HOW TO EAT YOUR W

A person starts on the road to illness the very first day his body burns up more energy than he is able to assimilate from his foods.

* * *

Dr. Reams believes one will never regain perfect health by treating effects. One must go to the cause.

* * *

Some people should never begin a health program with an immediate fast or light diet. There are specific guidelines one must follow to change your body chemistry.

* * *

There are good reasons why we should eat raw foods. And there are good reasons why one should not eat raw foods exclusively. It is important to know how to achieve the beneficial balance.

* * *

While coffee and tea are not recommended for a sound health program caution is advised in adapting a "change-over" diet to other liquids.

* * *

There are some foods you should avoid forever. Unfortunately many people include these foods in their basic diets.

* * *

A sound diet incorporates a balanced amount of "low stress" foods. There are several good reasons why "low stress" foods are necessary for vibrant health. Proper intake can increase both energy and endurance.

* * *

Meat should be well cooked. Rare meat should never be eaten. It is important to know how to prepare meat and how to trim fat.

* * *

High stress foods should never be a major part of your food intake!

* * *

Nature has provided us with sensible, valid ways to achieve inner peace. Never seek to secure this peace through a pill!

* * *

There is one basic reason why white potatoes should be eaten infrequently.

* * *

There is one excellent way to eliminate gas pains!

* * *

Nervous tension, insomnia and worry rob us of our joy and of our health. Proper food and liquid intake can go a long way to returning us to a vibrant life.

* * *

All this and much more you will find in **HOW TO EAT YOUR WAY BACK TO VIBRANT HEALTH.** Practical, step-by-step instructions for 7 weeks!

FOREWARD

I thank God for Salem Kirban and men like him who seek out truth, correlate it with the Bible, and publish it for everyone to read.

As a physician graduating in the late 40s, I received very little training in nutrition, as my branch of the healing arts deals mainly with detection and treatment of disease once it has become manifest.

My own interest in nutrition as a preventive for disease and maintenance of good health began when I was in Japan in 1956 in the military service. The diet there consisted almost exclusively of fresh vegetables and rice with fish as the meat. There was at that time very little high blood pressure, strokes or heart attacks. Now as their diet approaches ours, these diseases have rapidly increased in frequency!

Shortly after returning home I began to eat green salads, which I previously avoided, and more vegetables and less meat. I also began to eat only two meals a day, lunch around eleven in the morning and dinner around five o'clock in the afternoon. Yet something still seemed to be lacking.

About four years ago my wife, a registered nurse, began to feel depressed and with no energy. She sought medical advice and was given a mood elevating drug. When she realized what the drug was she became very upset as she felt this was not her problem. The Lord then led us to a book written by a minister and psychologist, part of which dealt with nutrition. My wife and I found our answer here and we both began to take food supplements, vitamins and minerals. My wife's depression soon left and she returned to her old vitality.

However, as we studied nutrition further we began to realize that we needed some guidance, the type of guidance as found in this book by Salem Kirban. In November, 1976, we had a Nutrition Profile Report prepared for us. Within a very short time we noticed a change in our health for the better. As we continue the program, we are adjusting our weights to the standard norms. Anytime we deviate from the prescribed regimen the next day we can feel the difference.

As I see my own patients and their difficulties, I become more convinced that a good many of our physical and mental problems are based on the present overall diet most of us eat. I am trying to guide my patients to a better diet and thus to better health.

The best answers to our problems, including diet, are found in the Bible and only when we return to God's Word for our guidance do we find true happiness.

Boude B. Leavel M.D.

SALEM KIRBAN
HOW TO EAT
Your Way Back To
VIBRANT HEALTH

HARVEST HOUSE PUBLISHERS Irvine, California 92714
Copyright © 1977 by Salem Kirban. Printed in the United States of America. All rights reserved, including the right to reproduce this book or portions thereof in any form.

ISBN 0-912582-25-1
Library of Congress Catalog Card No. 77-736-33

ACKNOWLEDGMENTS

To **Doreen Frick,** who carefully proofread the text.

To **Koechel Designs,** who designed the front cover.

To **Walter W. Slotilock,** Chapel Hill Litho, for skillfully making the illustration negatives.

To **Batsch Company, Inc.,** for excellent craftsmanship in setting the type quickly.

To **Bunn's Natural Food Shoppe,** for providing me with product information on health foods.

To **Dr. Carey Reams,** for giving me an abundant background of advice on nutrition.

To **Aunt Effie,** who contributed her opinions. Everyone has an Aunt Effie who thinks she knows the answer to every problem. You'll enjoy her old fashioned remedies but check them out with your doctor.

NOTE

The author is **not** a medical doctor. Nor is he posing as one! He is an investigative reporter. The author is interested in teaching the health message as found in the Bible.

The author makes no claims for a cure for any disease! Nor do we believe that drugs cure disease. Disease can only be corrected by the body's own healing and health-restoring power through God's grace.

We do not believe that the human body suffers from a deficiency of aspirin or a tranquilizer drug, etc. We do believe that most Americans are overfed and undernourished. We also believe that sound, intelligent nutrition practices are the first defense against disease and a better first alternative.

Nothing in this book, however, should imply to you that following this diet will solve your health problems. Nor do we in any way suggest you should put off seeking proper health advice from your doctor when the need arises.

It does cost money to maintain good health. But it costs much, much more to regain health once you have lost it!

DEDICATION

**To my wife
MARY**
Whose continual
faithful support
makes it possible
for me to write
with inspiration!

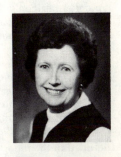

**To
Dr. CAREY REAMS**
Who showed me
how to live
and who taught me
the basics of nutrition
so I could
teach others!

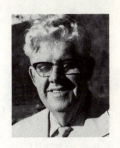

**To
Dr. JOHN L. BLACK**
who is carrying on the teaching program of Dr. Carey Reams.

**To
R. H. HOSKINS, Jr.**
who through the years has been Dr. Carey Reams' right hand man.

And to those dedicated men and women in the healing arts,
who without prejudice, are willing to use the information in this
book for the benefit of their patients — even if the truth happens
to be contrary to the prevailing orthodox thinking and practices.

WHY I WROTE THIS BOOK

In a recent report called "Dietary Goals for the United States," the Senate Select Committee on Nutrition and Human Needs concluded that we are eating our way into the hospital!

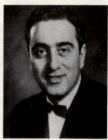

"*Numerous studies indicate that the typical American's diet may be as hazardous to his health as smoking,*" reports Committee Chairman Senator George McGovern.

Too much sugar, too much fat, or salt can be and are directly linked to heart disease, cancer, obesity and stroke, among other killer diseases. The Report observes that: "*Six of the 10 leading causes of death in the United States have been linked to our diet. Changing our diet is even more important to our health than national health insurance, and less costly in the long run.*"

Included in the report were specific guidelines to what the Committee considers a healthier diet:

1. Eat more fruit
2. Eat more vegetables and whole grains
3. Eat more poultry and fish

At the same time it recommended certain restrictions.

Not surprisingly, many of the committee's findings are unpalatable to the producers of cakes, pies, candies, soft drinks and processed meat products.

The costs for health care are rising at an astronomical rate. They take 10 cents out of every dollar of the average U.S. family's income. In the U.S., health care expeditures have tripled in the last 10 years! It is now over $140 billion! (This is over $2000 for an average family of 4). It is shocking to realize that **over 70%** of the annual American health bill of $140 billion goes for drugs, doctors, and hospitals. **Only 3%** goes for the prevention of disease!

The average cost per patient for a stay in a hospital was $311 in 1965. By 1974 it almost tripled to $873. Today it is well over $1000! But this does not tell the full story. The average individual's stay in a hospital is shorter now than it was 10 years ago . . . yet the expense per day is higher!

So many people after having read my book on Dr. Carey Reams, **HEALTH GUIDE FOR SURVIVAL**, wanted more information. This book, **HOW TO EAT YOUR WAY BACK TO VIBRANT HEALTH**, is a practical 7-Week Diet Plan which incorporates the essence of what Dr. Carey Reams recommends for a sound, nutritional diet.

Huntingdon Valley, Pennsylvania U.S.A., April, 1977

Salem Kirban

CONTENTS

Foreword by Boude B. Leavel, M.D. 2
Why I Wrote This Book 6
Nutrition ... A Better Alternative 8
The Salem Kirban 3-DAY TURN AROUND DIET 9
The Road to Good Health 13
Jerusalem (Jerusalem Jumpers) 14
Moses (Wilderness Wok) 15
Ezekiel (Ezekiel's Ecstasy) 16
Phoebe (Phoebe's Prune Delight) 17
Jacob (Jacob's Birthright Soup) 18
Elisheba (Elisheba's Eggplant Soup) 19
Caleb (Caleb's Carrot Soup) 20
Vashti (Vashti's Vegetable Soup) 21
Esther 22
Solomon (Solomon's Celery Soup) 24
Hagar (Hagar's Happening) 25
Abishag (Abishag's Casserole) 26
Dorcas (Dorcas's Dream Casserole) 27
Eve (Eve's Meatless Stew) 28
Gideon (Gideon's Gravy Gumbo) 29
Anna (Anna's Steamed Delight) 30
Rebekah (Rebekah's Raisin Pie) 31
Deborah (Deborah's Delight Cookies) 32
Dinah (Dinah's Date Bars) 33
Carob Chip Cookies 34
Raisin Molasses Bars 34
Reams' Review Soup 34
Week 1 35
Week 2 43
Week 3 51
Week 4 59
Week 5 67
Week 6 75
Week 7 83
Kirban's Cabbage Soup .... Color Insert
Salem's Salad (Tabbouleh) .... Color Insert
Esther's Stuffed Eggplant .... Color Insert
Index 91

NUTRITION... A BETTER ALTERNATIVE

Some people would rather die "*orthodox*" than live by "*unorthodox*" methods; namely, sound nutrition.

In one popular health column distributed by a newspaper syndicate, a medical doctor is asked: "*I would like to know how carrot juice and celery juice are good for the body?... Would it be okay to drink only carrot and celery juice for two days and not eat anything else in order to cleanse the system?*"

To which the doctor replied: "*You hear some weird medical claims for various foods and juices. Celery and carrot juice are harmless... but they have no magic qualities. I think that by now the quacks must have exhausted the supply of juices and foods they are always matching up with people's real ailments. Cleansing the system? You tell me what that means. How do you "cleanse" the human system? If researchers found a way to do it, I doubt it would be through carrot and celery juice....*"

It is difficult for some in the medical profession to accept sound nutritional guidelines as the first defense against disease. Fortunately, many doctors are now becoming nutrition conscious. The American Medical Association pinpoints the major cause of so many health problems: "*While much progress has been made in overcoming many historic plagues of mankind, we find more and more illness due, at least in part, to abuse and neglect by the individual himself.*"

Such an abuse by the individual most often occurs with a knife and fork. We eat the wrong foods. We drink the wrong liquids. Americans are well-fed and under-nourished.

It was Dr. Carey Reams, a noted biophysicist, who came to the conclusion that for every effect (bad health), there is a basic underlying cause (an unbalanced body chemistry). With 40 years of data and experience, Dr. Reams has successfully demonstrated the theory that health, good or bad, is the effect of diet and can be measured by mathematics.

Dr. Carey Reams is the discover of an ingenious **urine/saliva test**. This test yields the proper information to mathematically analyze the entire body chemistry. Dr. Reams states that heart attacks can be foreseen from minutes, to months, to years in advance — and prevented. **He also believes that cancer is caused because of lack of minerals!**

Based on the urine/saliva analysis, Dr. Reams is able to prepare a specific individualized diet designed to lead to excellent health. Mineral supplements are recommended on an individual basis to bring one's body chemistry back to normal. With proper body chemistry, Dr. Reams believes the body will heal itself. Incidentally, he is a firm believer in the use of carrot juice, celery juice and other live food juices. Dr. Reams, as do many others in the field of health, believe that nutrition is a far better and more rewarding alternative. After all, when you buy a carrot or a stalk of celery it is not labeled with a host of "side effects" and warnings.

The Salem Kirban
3-DAY TURN AROUND DIET

Perhaps, over the years, you have developed bad eating habits. You have emphasized fried foods, fish without scales (such as lobster, oysters, clams, shrimp), you have made a bonanza of desserts, cakes, pies and candies! You have minimized your intake of salads, fresh fruits and vegetables. And you have not been consistent in your water intake.

Perhaps now you feel a little rundown, fatigued. You may go to bed tired and wake up tired. Energy suddenly leaves you at 2 PM. You have trouble getting asleep and staying asleep. You are plagued with either diarrhea or constipation (or both)! You feel old at 23 or 34 or 44 or 58! You long for the days of your youth when you had vibrant energy and endurance. And you feel, perhaps, those days are gone forever. But are they? Many people your age have found the secret of vibrant health. And you can too.

This 3-Day Turn Around Diet is not a miracle plan. If you have been feeding the wrong fuel to your body over the years . . . don't expect it to turn around in 3 days. But, at least, these 3-days will set you on a course that should be beneficial. Many people can notice an immediate recognizable improvement in their well-being in this 3-Day Plan. They follow through on these 3 days by then following a sensible, nutritious diet. Of course there will be some days you will feel just plain miserable even in following a sound diet. It is a normal reaction as your body goes through withdrawal pains in flushing out the toxins.

As an example, if you are a heavy coffee drinker . . . don't give it up overnight. If you drink 6 cups a day . . . ease down over the period of a week or two to 3 cups a day and then the following week to 2 cups a day. Tea drinkers should follow the same advice. After a couple weeks of diminishing your intake of commercial teas . . . then start drinking herb teas.

As in any diet, you should first seek the advice of a doctor in whom you trust. Medication should NOT be discontinued during any diet plan unless your doctor specifically instructs you.

And then, above all, seek guidance and wisdom from the Great Physician. Enter into a diet with your mind free from the pressures of the day, the concerns, the worries that can do so much to undermine your health. And place these problems into the hands of God. **And LEAVE THEM THERE!**

ITEMS YOU WILL NEED	1 gallon Distilled Water 3 fresh Lemons 20-25 Carrots 2 stalks Celery 6 fresh Pears

You can purchase a gallon of distilled water in your local supermarket or drugstore. Make sure it says "distilled." Do not buy spring water or ionized water.

You will also need a **juicer**. For these 3 days you may possibly get by with a blender that would reduce the vegetables to a purée ... to which you could add some unsweetened pineapple juice. However, a juicer is preferred as this eliminates the pulp residues.

JUICE DELIGHT
Follow the below order of preparation. First:
    1 Pear (fresh) quartered and placed through juicer
Then add:
    1 single stalk Celery with leaves
Then add:
    Sufficient carrots to make 6 or 8 ounce glass requirement

JUICE of PEACE
Into juicer, place:
    3 stalks Celery with leaves
    Sufficient carrots to make 6 or 8 ounce glass requirement

    (If possible, run lettuce through your juicer to produce 1-2 ounces of lettuce juice and add to **JUICE of PEACE** combination)

Important
Do **NOT** make up juices ahead of time! Run them through your juicer right at the time you are ready to drink them. In this way you will capture most of the nutrients. Remember, green vegetables such as lettuce, celery, etc. ... **the greener they are** ... the higher the mineral content. If the carrots you buy seem bitter upon juicing ... they are no good. Carrots full of minerals and other nutrients are sweet tasting when reduced to juice. Try buying carrots that come from the West Coast or from a health food store.

DAY 1	**Breakfast**	Juice Delight (6 ounces) 1 Toast Hot herb tea or coffee
	Dinner	Fresh vegetable salad * 1 Toast (rye or cornbread) Juice Delight (6 ounces)
	Supper	Fresh vegetable salad * Celery soup Corn chips Juice of Peace (6 ounces)
		1 Yogurt before bedtime
DAY 2	**Breakfast**	Juice Delight (8 ounces) 1 Yogurt 1 Toast Hot herb tea or coffee
	Dinner	Fresh vegetable salad * Steamed carrots and green beans Juice Delight (8 ounces)
	Supper	Fresh vegetable salad * Celery soup 1 Toast Juice of Peace (8 ounces)
		1 Yogurt before bedtime
DAY 3	**Breakfast**	Juice Delight (8 ounces) 2 Eggs poached 1 Toast 1 Yogurt
	Dinner	Fresh vegetable salad * Vegetable Parade (Steamed carrots, onions, green beans and parsnips) 1 Toast Juice Delight (8 ounces)
	Supper	Vegetable soup Fresh vegetable salad * 1 Toast Juice of Peace (8 ounces)
		1 Yogurt before bedtime

* On your vegetable salad, be imaginative each day. Don't just use lettuce but include watercress, fresh parsley, endive, leeks, celery, spinach and carrot sticks, etc. Try olive oil as a dressing. And be sure to top off your salad with the juice of 1/2 freshly squeezed lemon.

Further Guidelines: Be sure to drink 4 ounces of distilled water every half hour as noted on next page. During these 3 days, don't watch television while in bed. Instead read a good book or a devotional or the Bible. If you normally retire 10:30, 11 or later at night... retire 1/2 hour to 1 hour earlier and relax by reading a little. Don't take your worries to bed! Rest in the Lord. *"Thou wilt keep him in perfect peace, whose mind is stayed on thee: because he trusteth in thee"* (Isaiah 26:3).

LIQUID INTAKE

On this 3-Day Turn Around Diet the key to its success lies in the consistent liquid intake. Most people do not drink sufficient liquids and do not drink it in the right quantity.

> Drink 4 ounces (no more and no less) of distilled water every 1/2 hour from 8 AM until 6 PM.
> Do not drink this distilled water 1/2 hour before your meal.
> Do not drink this distilled water during your meal.
> Do not resume drinking distilled water until 1/2 hour after your meal.

If you are drinking herb tea or coffee at mealtime, it is best to do so 1/2 hour after you have finished the meal.

MEDICINE

Confer with your doctor as to whether he believes it essential for you to continue medication while on this 3-day diet. Do not discontinue medication unless he tells you.

VITAMINS/MINERALS

If possible, do not take any during this 3-Day Turn Around Diet. If you do take them, vitamins should be taken between meals; minerals should be taken with meals.

ELIMINATION

Consistent bowel habits are important if one is to keep the toxins from building up in your system. Sluggishness, irritability, headaches are all possible indications of poor elimination habits. Many people find the pure herb Chaparral an excellent natural laxative that promotes daily elimination. Many health-minded people take 2 tablets (8.5 Grains) at each meal during this 3-Day Turn Around Diet.

FOLLOW-UP

After this 3-Day Turn Around Diet, you may wish to then pursue the **7-Week Diet** that follows in this book. If you choose this course, then resume the vitamin and mineral supplements you have been taking with your doctor's approval.

If you follow the **7-Week Diet Plan** you want to continue the 4-ounce distilled water intake every 1/2 hour, the same as recommended in the 3-Day Turn Around Diet program.

THE ROAD TO GOOD HEALTH

Mr. Kirban:
Is it possible to follow a sound nutritional program and still not achieve good health?

YES! You could follow the best advice medical doctors have to offer ... you could follow the best advice given by Dr. Reams and his associates ... you could faithfully follow a natural food diet, including drinking lemon water, distilled water and take the necessary minerals and vitamins. You could even fast. And still feel miserable!

Why? Because of your "whole being" attitude. It is believed that up to 80% of all illnesses are caused by our emotions and negative attitudes. And even though you follow all the rules for good health from a physical standpoint, yet have a poor mental attitude ... you still may not get results.

The road to good health includes (1) Spirit, (2) Soul and (3) Body (1 Thessalonians 5:23).

> **Spirit** (God-consciousness) is that part of man which "knows," his mind (1 Corinthians 2:11). Because man is a "spirit" he is capable of communication with God (Job 32:8; Psalm 18:28, Proverbs 20:27). Man's spirit is the spring of his inmost thoughts and intents (Numbers 5:14, Proverbs 16:18, Psalm 34:18).
>
> **Soul** implies a self-conscious life. Plants, as an example, have no soul. Our soul is the seat of our affections, desires, emotions and active will (Psalm 42:1-6).
>
> **Body** (world-consciousness) is the instrument or vehicle of the life of the soul (Deuteronomy 12:23, Isaiah 53:12; 2 Corinthians 5:10).

With this in mind, one can see that even though you feed the **body** properly and do all the right things nutritionally, yet have negative and critical attitudes, you will most likely not get results! The reason: your **spirit** and **soul,** because of your emotional attitudes, are starved, undernourished! As a result the whole being (including your body) suffers and illness often occurs (or continues)!

Specifically, in over 2000 case histories I have observed, where Nutrition Profiles have been recommended, I have met people who are more interested in knowing what their ailments are rather than adopting a nutritional program for better health. They prefer to dwell on their disease; comparing laboratory numbers and becoming engulfed in medical terminology. Their entire mental attitude is wrong. Their soul and spirit are sick. And regardless how religiously they follow a nutritional program ... they most likely will never get satisfactory results until they align spirit, soul and body into a positive harmony! Negative emotions can produce a stagnant pool. A happy, positive balance of Spirit, Soul and Body can produce a gentle flowing river!
The choice is yours!

JERUSALEM

Name Means: City of Peace.

Jerusalem has a recorded history of some 4000 years. It has been more familiar to more people for a longer period than any other place on earth. It was known (about 1400 B.C.) as U-ru-sa-lim which means "city of Salim."

Jerusalem stands in the center of Israel, some 40 miles inland from the Mediterranean coast. This is the city of David, who in the 10th century B.C. unified the country and proclaimed Jerusalem the capital. This is the city of Solomon's Temple and where Isaiah and Jeremiah prophesied.

Jerusalem stands at the head of no great river. It overlooks no great harbor. It commands no great highway nor crossroads. It is not close to an abundant source of water. It possesses no mineral riches. And yet, Jerusalem has risen to unequalled greatness!

Jerusalem is called the city of God (Psalms 46:4; 48:1,8; 87:3; Hebrews 12:22 and Revelation 3:12). Jerusalem was destroyed by Nebuchadnezzar in 587 B.C. It was controlled by Alexander the Great (332 B.C.) and conquered by Pompey (63 A.D.). It fell to Titus in 70 A.D. and was totally destroyed by Hadrian in 135 A.D. The Persians captured Jerusalem in 614 A.D.; the Byzantines recaptured the city in 629 A.D. The Crusaders captured Jerusalem in 1099 A.D. And Saladin recaptured the city in 1187 A.D. In 1517 it fell to the Ottoman empire and in 1917 the British conquest occurred. Finally, in May, 1948 the State of Israel was proclaimed. It has been said that more wars have been fought over Jerusalem than any other city!

> Ten portions of beauty
>   descended to the world,
> Jerusalem acquired nine
>   The rest of the world, one.
> Ten portions of suffering
>   descended to the world,
> Jerusalem acquired nine
>   The rest of the world, one.

JERUSALEM JUMPERS
About 12   4-Inch Cakes

Measure and place in a bowl:
- **1 cup cornmeal (white or yellow)**
- **2 tablespoons honey**
- **1 teaspoon sea salt**

Stir in slowly:
- **1 cup boiling distilled water**

Cover this mixture. Let stand 10 minutes. Beat in separate bowl:
- **1 egg**
- **1/2 cup milk**
- **2 tablespoons melted butter**

Add these to the cornmeal mixture. Then add sifted:
- **1/2 cup flour**

Resift with:
- **2 teaspoons double-acting baking powder**

Stir ingredients into the batter using a few swift strokes.

Tips on Making Pancakes:
Don't overbeat. Just give enough quick strokes to moisten the dry ingredients. Don't worry about lumps. Best results are obtained when pancake batter is quickly mixed and then rested. Allow to sit in refrigerator for 3-6 hours before using. If batter is too thick, add a little water; if too thin, add a little flour. Make sure griddle is hot (water drops should bounce off!). Let batter pour from tip of your spoon on to griddle to get well-rounded cake. It will be 2-3 minutes before cake is ready to turn. When bubbles appear on top surface (but before they break), turn pancake over. Turn the cake only once! Second side takes half as long to cook.

MOSES
The deliverer of Israel

Name Means: Drawn out.
Family: Son of Amram and Jochebed
Scripture: Exodus, Numbers, Deuteronomy

Moses was a great Hebrew leader. He was born at the time the king of Egypt was determined to destroy every newly born male child among the Israelites. He was rescued from the water, where his mother had hid him, by Pharaoh's daughter. Moses lived 120 years. This was divided into three sections of 40 years each.

The first 40 years -
   Pharaoh's son
The second 40 years -
   In the desert
The third 40 years -
   Leading the Israelites

Moses led some 600,000 men plus women and children through the wilderness. The Israelites arrived at Kadesh within two years and were in sight of the Promised Land. Afraid to enter, they turned back. Their wilderness walk lasted another 38 years! Sin crept into the camp. They grumbled about the food and yearned for the leeks and garlic of Egypt (Numbers 11:4,5). God sent them quails and they made gluttons of themselves and got sick (Numbers 11:33). God sent them Manna from heaven and they growled again (Num. 21:5).

Moses saw the Promised Land but never entered it. He died with perfect eyesight and in full vigor at the ripe age of 120 on Mt. Nebo (Deuteronomy 34:6).

* A play on words for "walk." Since this menu has a Chinese origin, it is suggested that a Wok be used if you have one. A Wok is a metal cooking pan with a convex bottom and is often used for frying or steaming.

WILDERNESS WOK *
6 Servings

Sear in Wok or skillet:
   1 onion diced
Add:
   1 cup long-grain rice
Then add:
   whipped eggs (2 per serving)
Cook slowly until rice grains separate and are tender. Season to taste with vegetable seasonings.

Tips on Rice:
Brown rice retains its bran coat and germ and is much slower to tenderize. However it is more valuable nutritionally than highly polished white rice.

Long-grain rice is best where you desire each grain to be separate and fluffy. Generally, 1 cup of raw rice yields 3 cups when cooked.

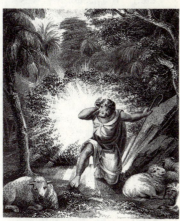

In the midst of the burning bush, God calls Moses and promises to deliver the Israelites from Egypt's oppression to a land flowing with milk and honey (Exodus 3:1-8).

EZEKIEL
The watchman for Israel

Name Means: God strengthens.
Family: The son of Buzi, a priest
Scripture: The book of Ezekiel

Ezekiel grew up in Judea during its last years of independence. He was deported to Babylon with Jehoiachin, King of Judah, in 597 B.C. when Ezekiel was but 25 years old. For 11 years, 10,000 exiles lived in this strange country. For five years they had no preacher. Then Ezekiel accepted the call and tried to warn them of a long exile and the coming destruction of Jerusalem. Jeremiah lived in Jerusalem during this time. Ezekiel and Daniel both lived in Babylon. However, Ezekiel lived with the exiles while Daniel lived in Nebuchadnezzar's court.

Ezekiel was a powerful preacher. His favorite expression was: "The hand of the Lord was upon me" (see Ezekiel 1:3, 3:14, 22 etc.). His preaching was often resented because it was forthright. Ezekiel pronounced doom on Judah's enemies (Ezekiel 25-32). He reminds them that they benefited by trading with Judah and the land of Israel. Among the items traded were Millet, known in Bible days as Pannag or the wheat of Minneth. Millet was used to make a good grade of flour, its seeds being hard and white. One stalk may carry a thousand grains!

Ezekiel, in a vision, sees a great valley, filled with dry bones, which suddenly come to life (Ezekiel 37:11-14). This prophetically foretells the restoration of the whole house of Israel.

EZEKIEL'S ECSTASY (Millet)
4 Servings

It is best to presoak millet for 48 hours in a covered container.

To cook, use:
  3-4 cups skim milk
for every:
  1 cup dry cereal
Cook covered for 45 minutes to 1 hour until translucent and tender.
Mix in:
  raisins
  honey
  allspice
to taste.

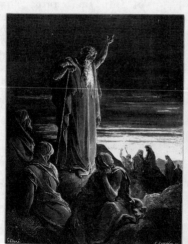

Ezekiel envisions the restoration of Israel (Ezekiel 37:11-14).

PHOEBE
The woman who served

Name Means: Pure and radiant.
Identification: A deaconess in the early Christian church.
Scripture Reference: Romans 16:1,2

Phoebe was one of the first woman helpers in the early Christian church. She served at Cenchrea at the port of Corinth when Paul arrived there at the end of his third journey. It was here Paul wrote his letter to the Romans. Paul urged those in Rome to "... *receive her in the Lord in a manner worthy of the saints, and that you help her in whatever matter she may have need of you; for she herself has also been a helper of many, and of myself as well*" (Romans 16:2).

Phoebe was both faithful and a friend in need ... always willing to lend a helping hand as part of her faithful service.

PHOEBE'S PRUNE DELIGHT

48 hours in advance of use, soak:

3 prunes (per person)

in Lemon Water to cover in refrigerator.

Lemon Water is one part fresh Lemon juice to *nine* parts of distilled water. Serve in bowl on Graham crackers.

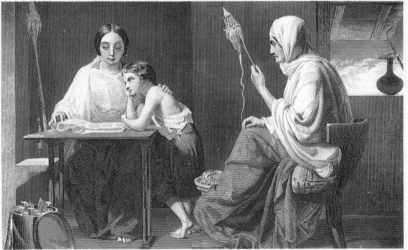

Phoebe faithfully served in Corinth. At the height of its power, Corinth probably had a free population of 200,000, plus a half million slaves. Corinth was a city of wealth, luxury and immorality.

JACOB
Father of 12 tribes of Israel

Name Means: He that followeth after.
Identification: The second son of Isaac and Rebekah.
Scripture References: Genesis 25-49

Jacob was his mother's first love although he was Rebekah's second son, Isaac favored Esau, the hunter. Jacob and Esau were twin brothers. Esau, being born first, would normally become the inheritor of Isaac's death-bed blessing.

One day, Jacob was boiling a lentil stew. Lentils were a popular dish in Bible days because of their abundance and high protein value.

Esau, returning from a hunting trip, was famished, ready to faint, and begged Jacob for some of the lentil stew. Jacob made a bargain: *"First sell me your birthright"* (Genesis 25:31). Esau, so desperately hungry, agreed. It was the beginning of a bitter feud.

When Isaac was about to die his wife Rebekah schemed with Jacob to dress in Esau's skins and fool his father into passing on the blessing to him. Rebekah was never to see her son Jacob again!

Esau was furious and Jacob fled to Haran. It was the beginning of a bloody feud that would cost countless lives throughout succeeding centuries.

It was Herod (of Esau's race) who had the male infants of Bethlehem slain in an effort to destroy the Christ child.

JACOB'S BIRTHRIGHT Soup
6 Servings

Wash well and drain:
- 2 **cups lentils (split red)**

Add:
- 10 **cups boiling water**
- 1 **marrow bone cracked**

Simmer about 4 hours. During last hour, add:
- 1 **large onion chopped and sautéed in 3 tablespoons butter**
- 1 **stalk celery with leaves chopped**
- 2 **carrots chopped**
- 2 **garlic cloves minced**

Before serving, blend in:
- Juice of 1 lemon
- Health food seasonings

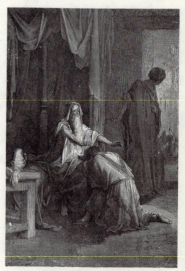

Isaac blesses Jacob.

ELISHEBA
Mother of Levitical priesthood

Name Means: God is her oath.
Identification: Wife of Aaron, the high priest.
Scripture Reference: Exodus 6:23

Elisheba probably was born towards the close of the bondage in Egypt. No doubt she witnessed the results of the cruel edict of Pharoah for the destruction of male children. She was a sister of Naashon who was the leader of the tribe of Judah on the march through the wilderness.

She married Aaron the high priest. Aaron was the brother of Moses. This marriage made her a part of the royal and priestly tribes.

Elisheba gave birth to Nadab, Abihu, Eleazar and Ithamar. And by so doing, she became the foundress of the entire Levitical priesthood.

ELISHEBA'S EGGPLANT SOUP
6 Servings

In heavy bottom pot, heat:
- **2 tablespoons olive oil**
- **2 tablespoons butter**

Add and sauté:
- **1 onion chopped**

Then add:
- **1 eggplant diced**
- **2 cloves garlic mashed**
- **1/2 cup carrots chopped**
- **1/2 cup celery chopped**
- **1 large can (1 lb., 12 oz.) pear-shaped tomatoes** (Break up tomatoes with knife or fork)
- **2 cans (14 oz.) beef broth**
- **1/2 teaspoon honey**
- **1/2 teaspoon allspice**
- **1/8 teaspoon cayenne pepper**

Cover and simmer for about 30 minutes.

Add:
- **1/2 cup vegetable macaroni**
- **2 tablespoons parsley**

Simmer 10 minutes more or until macaroni is tender. For added touch, sprinkle cheese over each serving.

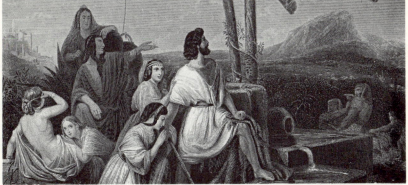

The women gather around Moses as he surveys the results of the successful war of the Israelites against the Midianites (Numbers 31).

CALEB
The man who desired a mountain

Name Means: Bold, impetuous.
Identification: One of chief spies sent out by Moses.
Scripture References: Numbers, Joshua, Judges

Caleb, at 40 years of age, represented his tribe and was among the twelve men that Moses sent from the wilderness to Paran to spy out the Promised Land. See Numbers 13:6. Of the 12 spies, 10 came back with a pessimistic report saying: "... *we saw the giants, the sons of Anak ... and we were in our own sight, as grasshoppers, and so we were in their sight"* (Numbers 13:33). Many people today have a "grasshopper" complex when faced with situations that seem difficult. They back down and make excuses.

Caleb and Joshua brought back a favorable report of the Promised Land. Caleb urged: "... <u>let us go up at once, and possess it; for we are well able to overcome it"</u> **(Numbers 13:30)**.

Because the people of Israel, in cowardice, adopted the majority report, God made them wander a total of 40 years in the wilderness. For Caleb's faithfulness, at the age of 85, he was given the area that is now Hebron.

CALEB'S CARROT SOUP
10 Servings

Sauté briefly in:
   2 tablespoons butter
with enough water to cover:
   4-6 carrots chopped (1½ lbs.)
Add:
   1/2 teaspoon honey
   Vegetable seasoning to taste
Bring to boil, cover pan and simmer until carrots are soft. Then drain and mash carrots to a purée (or use electric blender). Combine carrot purée with:
   7½ cups chicken stock
Bring to boil and simmer gently until purée has dissolved
Melt in a separate pan:
   3 tablespoons butter
Add and blend slowly:
   2½ tablespoons flour
Gradually over low heat add:
   1/2 cup milk
and cook until this thickens. Then remove from heat and add:
   3 egg yolks
one at a time, beating constantly. Then add this mixture to soup, mixing vigorously. Adjust seasoning. Bring to boiling point for a second. Then remove from heat and serve.

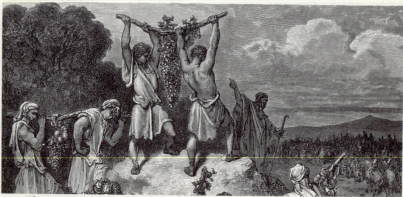

The spies return with grapes from the Valley of Eshcol. (Numbers 13:23).

VASHTI
The woman who withstood a king

Name Means: Beautiful woman.
Identification: Queen of the court of Ahasurerus (Xerxes)
Scripture References: Esther 1; 2:1; 4:17

Vashti, by birth, was a Persian princess. Her husband, King Ahasurerus, reigned from India to Ethiopia over 127 provinces from 486 to 465 B.C. The King was an absolute monarch who exercised unlimited authority over the life and death of his subjects.

In order to impress the princes and nobles of his power, he called them to Susa, the capital of Persia. They were to be entertained for 180 days! Following this 180 days, the King prepared a great feast which was to last seven days. Nothing was spared. The main hall was decorated with rich awnings; the reclining couches for the guests were of gold and silver (Esther 1:6). Drinks were served in golden goblets (Esther 1:7).

By the seventh day of the banquet the King was drunk. He summoned Vashti his wife to appear in the banquet hall unveiled. This was against all Persian custom for a woman to be displayed before an audience even in regal robes.

Queen Vashti, standing firm in her modesty, refused the King's request. The King was enraged and he issued a decree: "... *let it be written among the laws of the Persians and Medes so that it may not be changed, that Vashti is to be divorced ...* (Esther 1:19).

Vashti chose Christian ideals in womanhood rather than dishonor.

VASHTI'S VEGETABLE SOUP
4 Servings

Sauté briefly in heavy bottom pot:
- 1/4 cup carrots diced
- 1/2 cup onions diced
- 1/2 cup celery diced

Add:
- 3 cups soup stock
- 1 bay leaf
- 1 cup canned tomatoes
- 1/2 cup turnips diced
- 1 tablespoon parsley

Season to taste with vegetable seasonings. Cover and simmer for about 35 minutes; then add:
- 1/2 cup spinach chopped

Cook about 5 minutes more.

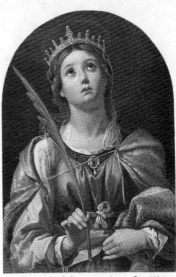

Vashti stood firm against the King.

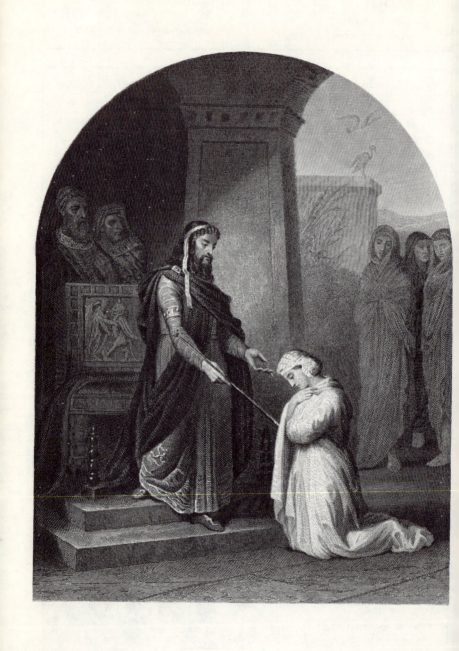

ESTHER
The Woman who saved her Nation

Name Means: A star.
Family: Queen of Persia
Scripture: The Book of Esther

Esther was a Jewish orphan maiden in the city of Shushan, the Persian royal city. Her Hebrew name was Hadassah which means *myrtle*. Her cousin, Mordecai, was a minor official of the palace under Xerxes, the Persian king. Mordecai raised Esther as his own daughter. She had a striking, personal beauty.

When Xerxes, having divorced his wife Vashti, sought a new queen, he asked that all fair maidens come to his harem for the selection process. Each maiden went through a 12 month beauty school (Esther 2:12). For six months they were beautified with oil of myrrh and another six months with sweet spices and perfumes.

At the end of the selection process Xerxes (King Ahasuerus) chose Esther to be his queen. The king also made Haman, an enemy of the Jews, his chief minister. Everybody bowed down to Haman except Mordecai. This infuriated Haman and in revenge he sought to destroy all the Jews (Esther 3:6). Lots, called Pur, were cast to decide on a day for this destruction.

Mordecai urged Esther to appear before the King and plead the cause of the people of the Hebrew race. She appeared at a banquet and suggested another banquet meeting where Haman would also be a guest. Haman, self-assured, had a gallows constructed on which to hang Mordecai. That night the King could not sleep and so he asked that the royal chronicles be read him. In these chronicles he discovered that Mordecai had uncovered an assasination plot and had saved the King's life ... yet Mordecai had not received any reward for this action.

At the second banquet, Esther pointed the finger at Haman as the one responsible for the threat of death to her people. The King was infuriated at Haman's action for he realized that Mordecai had saved the King's life. He ordered Haman hanged from the very gallows that Haman had constructed for Mordecai.

On the day when the massacre was to take place, the Jews and their friends, were victorious in the two-day battle. Over 75,000 of the enemy were killed. Esther and Mordecai wrote letters to the Jews to mark these two days as a Feast of Purim (Esther 9:21).

Esther was known as the woman who saved her nation from extermination. Would that an Esther was present during World War 2!

(Esther's Stuffed Eggplant recipe is found in the color section in the center of this book.)

SOLOMON
The man who asked for wisdom

Name Means: Peaceable.
Identification: Son of David and Bathsheba.
Scripture References: 2 Samuel, 1 Chronicles, 1 Kings

Solomon was born with all the advantages that one could ever wish for. His father, David, had immense stores of wealth and he was to occupy his father's throne as King.

Solomon was made king when he was 19. His kingdom of 60,000 square miles was ten times as great as that which his father had inherited! Realizing his responsibility, he sought the Lord. In a dream by night, God said, *"Ask what I shall give thee"* (1 Kings 3:5). Solomon asked that he might have wisdom to judge the people and to discern between good and bad (1 King 3:9). God granted his wish providing he would walk *". . . in My ways, to keep my statutes and my commandments"* (1 Kings 3:12-14).

Solomon's fame and fortune were known throughout the world. In one year his income in gold alone was $19,980,000! (This was pre-inflation days!) The Queen of Sheba, hearing of his fame, went to see for herself and remarked: *"I believed not the words, until I came, and mine eyes had seen it: and, behold, the half was not told me: thy wisdom and prosperity exceedeth the fame which I heard"* (1 Kings 10:7).

Solomon's greatest undertaking was the building of the Temple. Taxes become so heavy they weighed the people down. Their morale was broken because of luxury and idolatry. Solomon began a series of marriage alliances which eventually became his undoing. He surrounded himself with 700 wives and 300 concubines (1 Kings 11:3). He reigned for 40 years and died in 930 B.C.

SOLOMON'S CELERY SOUP
6 Servings

Sauté briefly in heavy skillet:
  1 tablespoon butter
  1 onion chopped
  2 cups celery chopped
  1 tablespoon flour
Transfer to soup pot and add:
  4 cups chicken soup stock
  (or chicken broth)
Simmer until celery is tender and then add:
  1½ cups light cream
Sprinkle with parsley and serve.

For added nutrition and zest include 1 cup of eggplant diced.

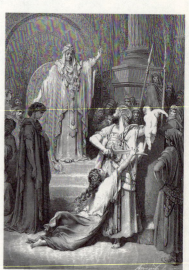

Solomon exercised wisdom in determining which woman was the mother of the baby (1 Kings 3:16-28).

HAGAR
The mother of Arab nations

Name Means: Flight
Identification: Handmaid to Sarah
Scripture References: Genesis 16; 21:9-17; 25:12; Galatians 4:24, 25

Hagar was the mother of the Arab peoples. She was an Egyptian handmaid to Sarah, wife of Abraham. God had promised Abraham a son who would be his heir. However, Sarah bore no children. Following the marital customs of the day, Sarah gave Hagar to her husband so that a son could be born. Sarah ran ahead of God and because of this trouble occurred.

Hagar, realizing she was pregnant, despised Sarah (Genesis 16:4). Sarah, engulfed in rivalry, scorned Hagar to the point where Hagar finally fled the household and went into the wilderness.

The angel of the Lord promised Hagar: *"I will multiply your descendants exceedingly so that they shall not be numbered for multitude"* (Genesis 16:10). Hagar returned to the household and gave birth to Ishmael *(God hears).* Ishmael was born when Abraham was 86 years old.

When Ishmael was 14 and Abraham was 100, Sarah gave birth to Isaac at age 90. Ishmael scoffed at Isaac. This infuriated Sarah and she demanded that Hagar and Ishmael leave the household (Genesis 21:10). Abraham, with love and concern, arose early the next morning and gave Hagar bread and a bottle of water and bid them goodbye. Hagar wandered aimlessly with Ishmael in the wilderness of Beersheba and soon the water was gone. She pleaded with the Lord, weeping that she not have to witness the death of her son from lack of food. God spoke to her saying: *"Arise . . . I intend to make him a great nation"* (Genesis 21:18). Hagar is last seen taking for her son a wife. Ishmael died at the age of 137. And the rivalry between Arab and Jew has run through oceans of blood that still have not been quenched.

HAGAR'S HAPPENING Casserole
6 Servings

Soak overnight:
  1 cup lentils

Drain soaked lentils and simmer in large pot in 2½ cups water for about 1 hour. Add:
  2 potatoes diced
  1/2 lb. zucchinni cubed
  1/2 lb. leeks chopped
  1 stalk celery chopped
  1/2 cup mushrooms
  Vegetable seasoning to taste

Simmer 15-20 minutes, adding more water if necessary.

Fry:
  1 onion finely chopped
until transparent. Then add:
  2 cloves garlic crushed
and fry for a minute or two longer. Drain and add to the lentils and vegetables together with:
  2 tablespoons parsley chopped
  Juice of 2 fresh lemons

Simmer for a few minutes and serve.

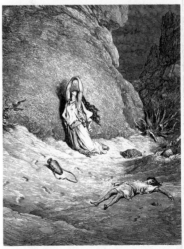

Hagar pleads for God's mercy.

ABISHAG
The woman who nursed a king

Name Means: My father wanders or errs.
Identification: She was a Shunamitess from Issachar.
Scripture References: 1 Kings 1:3,4; 2:13-25

Abishag was the woman who nursed King David in his old age. David was 70. He had but a few more months to live. Because of his feebleness and his inability to keep warm, his physicians suggested they secure the services of a young maiden to be his nurse. They searched over entire Israel and finally selected Abishag, a beautiful Shunammite girl.

There was no marital relationship. Abishag became the practical nurse for a dying King. Undoubtedly she helped prepare many life-sustaining meals.

ABISHAG'S Casserole
6 Servings

Oven:
Preheat oven to 350° F.
In large skillet, sauté gently until tender (about 10 minutes). Do not brown.
- 1 **cup celery diced**
- 2 **cups carrots, sliced**
- 1 **onion (medium) chopped**
- 3 **tablespoons oil**

Add seasonings to sautéed vegetables:
- 1/2 **cup blanched shredded almonds**
- 1/8 **teaspoon cayenne**
- 1/4 **teaspoon rosemary**
- 3 **teaspoons parsley**
- 1 **teaspoon mint**

Remove to 2 quart casserole and add and stir thoroughly:
- 2 **cups tomato purée**
- 2 **cups distilled water**

Bake in preheated oven for 45 minutes. Check occasionally to see if additional liquid is required. For additional flavor you may add 1 cup of beef broth. If you add beef broth, only use 1 cup of distilled water.

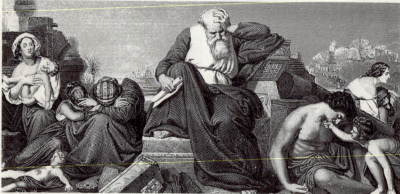

David, in his old age, had much opportunity to reflect on both his trials and his triumphs. The building of the Temple would be left to Solomon.

DORCAS
The dressmaker who served

Name Means: Gazelle
Identification: An early Christian disciple.
Scripture Reference: Acts 9:36-43

Dorcas lived in the seaport town of Joppa (now Jaffa). She became known for her many acts of charity during the time of the early Christian Church.

When she died the whole church mourned her passing. Some of her friends learned that Peter was nearby. Two members were dispatched to plead with him to visit the sorrowing church members in Joppa.

Peter arrived and was moved by their compassion for this woman who had unselfishly given her time and talents to benefit others. Peter asked them to leave the room, He knelt down, prayed. Then, with the power given him by God, he bade Dorcas to arise. Quickly she got up and Peter presented her to her friends in the next room.

The raising of Dorcas brought about a revival "... *and many came to believe on the Lord*" (Acts 9:42).

DORCAS'S DREAM Casserole
8 Servings

Peel, slice and dry on paper towel
    2½ cups eggplant diced and set aside.
Put in deep skillet:
    1/3 cup olive oil
Sauté until golden
    1 cup onions diced
    3 cloves garlic diced
    4 green peppers diced
    3 cups zucchini "1/2" slices
    2 cups quartered tomatoes
Add:
    eggplant
Sprinkle top with olive oil
Add:
    2 teaspoons basil
    1 teaspoon allspice

Simmer covered over very low heat for about 45 minutes. Uncover and continue heat 15 minutes to reduce liquid. Season to taste with vegetable seasonings.

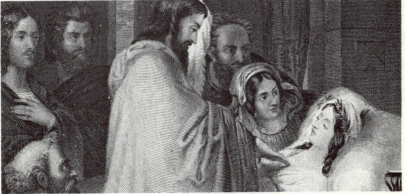
Through God's power, a miracle was performed in the life of Dorcas.

EVE
The first companion

Name Means: Mother of all living.
Identification: Adam's wife.
Scripture References: Genesis 2 and 3; 2 Corinthians 11:3; 1 Timothy 2:13

Eve, initially, was a complete, perfect woman. God fashioned Eve out of a bone taken from Adam's side. She was never a child. Eve was the first woman to live upon the earth and she was the first woman to be called a wife. She became man's counterpart and companion. Eve was the first and only woman born without sin.

Tempted by Satan to eat of the fruit of the tree in the Garden of Eden, Eve succumbed, believing she would be made more wise. Because she disobeyed God, women from that day on would suffer during pregnancy and labor.

Eve became the first dressmaker, the first mother to have a son who was a murderer (Cain). Adam and Eve both lived approximately 930 years!

EVE'S MEATLESS STEW
6 Servings

Sauté in skillet:
    3 tablespoons olive oil
    1 clove garlic chopped
   12 small onions
Transfer above to heavy bottom pot and add:
    1 cup distilled water
    3 cups beef broth
    2 bay leaves
    4 carrots sliced
    1 small turnip diced
    4 small potatoes diced
    1 cup okra chopped

Simmer for one hour or until vegetables are tender but firm. Season to taste. To thicken dissolve potato or rye flour (3-4 tablespoons) in 1/2 cup cold water, stirring until smooth, then adding to stew.

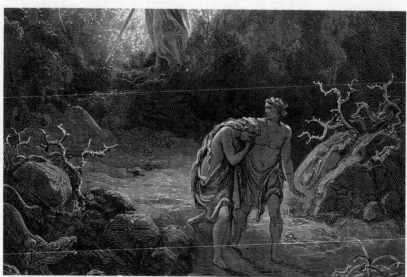

Adam and Eve are turned away from the Garden of Eden.

GIDEON
The man of might and valor

Name Means: To hew or cut down.
Identification: Delivered Israel from the Midianites.
Scripture Reference: The Book of Judges; Hebrews 11:32

Gideon, although he came from a poor family, accepted the call of the Lord and released the people of Israel from seven years of bondage under the Midianites. Everyone remembers how Gideon sought God's leading by placing a fleece of wool on the floor and asking for a sign of assurance. God gave Gideon the assurance that he would be victorious.

He prepared to go to battle against the Midianites. It has been estimated that the Midianites had a host of more than 135,000 soldiers and possibly 300,000! Gideon had 32,000 men. God wanted Gideon and the Israelites to exercise faith and not to conquer the Midianites in their own strength because such a victory might bring pride (Judges 7:2). Through a series of tests, the army was pared down to just 300 men. The 31,700 were sent home. Think of it! 300 men against possibly 300,000! But God had made a promise that 100 could put 10,000 to flight (Leviticus 26:8). With God on our side . . . **ONE is a MAJORITY!** Gideon obeyed God's directions and:

1. Divided the 300 men into 3 companies.
2. Put a trumpet into the hand of every man with an empty pitcher and a lamp burning in the pitcher.
3. Directed the 300 to surround the camp. Then they broke the pitchers and held the lamps in their left hand and shouted THE SWORD OF THE LORD AND OF GIDEON!

The breaking of the pitchers, the sounding of the trumpets, the eerie lamps burning in the middle of the night, frightened the soldiers. They panicked and began slaying each other in the confusion. Gideon pursued them all the way to juncture of the Sea of Galilee and the Jordan River. Gideon refused the offer of his people to become king but served for 40 years as judge (Judges 8:28).

GIDEON'S GRAVY GUMBO
4 Servings

Sauté until browned
  1 onion chopped
in butter and add:
  2 cups whole milk
    gluten flour sufficient to thicken mixture
  1 egg whipped
    vegetarian ham chopped
Cook and stir well. You may wish to add Gravy Master or Kitchen Bouquet.

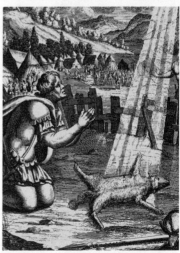

Gideon seeks God's will through a fleece. God promises to deliver Israel (Judges 6:36-40).

ANNA
The woman with a singular message

Name Means: Favor or Grace
Identification: Daughter of Phanuel of tribe of Asher.
Scripture References: Luke 2:36-38

Anna, widowed after seven years of marriage, became a prophetess. At the age of 84, when the infant Jesus was brought into the Temple to be dedicated, she recognized Him and proclaimed Him as the Messiah.

Anna never left the Temple but served there both day and night in prayer and fasting. Her entire life was focused on this one great event . . . that of identifying and proclaiming Jesus Christ as Messiah.

ANNA'S STEAMED DELIGHT
4 Servings

Place sufficient water in pot and allow it to boil briskly. Then place on perforated top the following vegetables:

2 cups carrots diced
1 onion diced
2 potatoes cubed
4 parsnips chopped

Place perforated top into steaming pot and cook until tender. Remove and add the juice of one lemon.

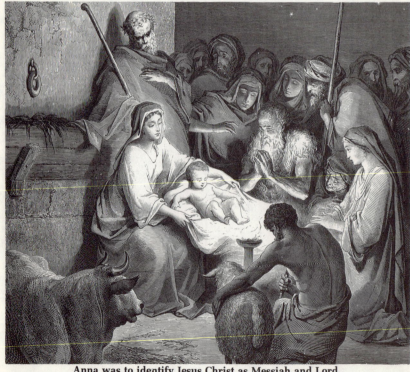

Anna was to identify Jesus Christ as Messiah and Lord.

REBEKAH
The Woman with great desires

Name Means: Captivating.
Identification: Wife of Isaac.
Scripture Reference: Genesis 22-49:21; Romans 9:6-16

Rebekah's grandfather was Nahor, Abraham's brother (Genesis 22:20-24). Nahor had a son, Bethuel, who became the father of Rebekah.

The love story of Rebekah and Isaac is a poignant one. Eliezer, a servant, was dispatched by Abraham to seek a bride for Isaac. Eliezer met Rebekah at a well and saw that she was very beautiful and attractive (Genesis 24:16). He went to Rebekah's brother, Laban, and asked permission to present Rebekah to Isaac. Laban consented (Genesis 24:51).

Isaac was 40 years old when he married Rebekah and they loved each other. But for twenty years they had no children. Then Isaac prayed asking the Lord to grant them children (Genesis 25:21). And God answered their prayer. Twins were born. Esau arrived first and then Jacob.

Jacob became his mother's favorite. Rebekah and Jacob deceived aging Isaac into bestowing the blessing to Jacob rather than Esau, the first born. Jacob had to flee from his home because of Esau's anger.

It was the last time Rebekah saw her son. Rebekah was buried in the cave of Machpelah in Hebron.

REBEKAH'S RAISIN PIE
One 9-inch Pie

Preheat oven to 375°.
Soak raisins in water until plump.
In medium-size pan, mix:

- 1 egg beaten
- 1/3 cup honey

Add:
- 1 cup soaked raisins
- 4 tablespoons lemon juice
- 1 teaspoon grated lemon rind

Cook over medium heat and add:
- 2 tablespoons cornstarch which has been dissolved in
- 1/2 cup distilled water

Continue cooking until raisin filling is thickened. Then allow mixture to cool. Fill pie shell. Bake in 9-inch pie pan in 375° preheated oven for 1/2 hour.

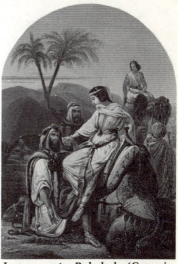

Isaac meets Rebekah (Genesis 24:64).

DEBORAH
The woman who served

Name Means: Bee
Identification: Rebekah's nurse.
Scripture Reference: Genesis 24:59; 35:8

Deborah accompanied Rebekah to her new home after her marriage to Isaac. She helped raise Jacob and Esau. When Rebekah's children reached adulthood she did not dispense of Deborah but included her as part of their family because of her faithfulness.

Great honor was paid to her when she died at a very old age. She was buried under an oak tree whose name Jacob called *Allon-bachuth* (which means, Oak of Weeping).

Another Deborah in Scripture was one of Israel's judges (Judges 4 and 5), a woman who became a fearless patriot.

DEBORAH'S DELIGHT Cookies
About 5 Dozen

Preheat oven to 350°.
Mix together and beat well:
  2/3 **cup honey**
  1/2 **cup oil**
  1 **egg**
Then stir in:
  4 **tablespoons molasses**
  1 **teaspoon cinnamon**
  1 **teaspoon ginger**
  2 **cups flour** *
  2 **teaspoons baking soda**

Drop batter by the teaspoonful into 1/4 cup cinnamon/flour **or** allspice/flour mixture. Form into balls. Place coated balls on cookie sheet about 3 inches apart. Bake for 8-10 minutes.

* Add sufficient to achieve cookie dough consistency.

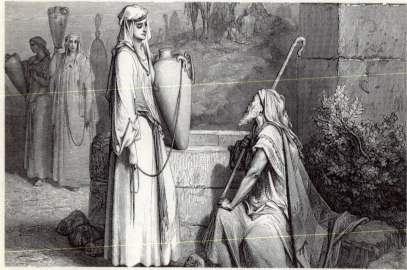

Deborah faithfully served Rebekah for many years.

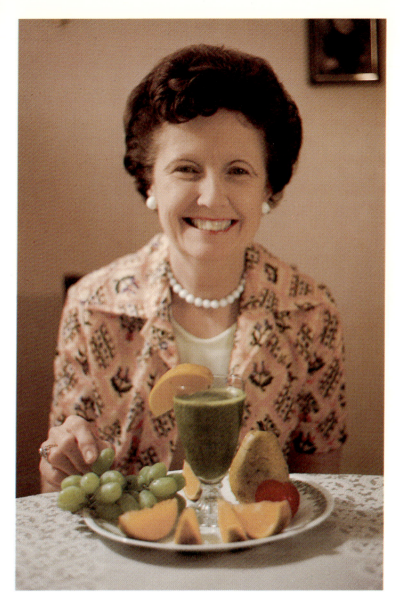

My wife, Mary, displays an attractive fruit platter. In the center is Green Drink topped with an orange slice.

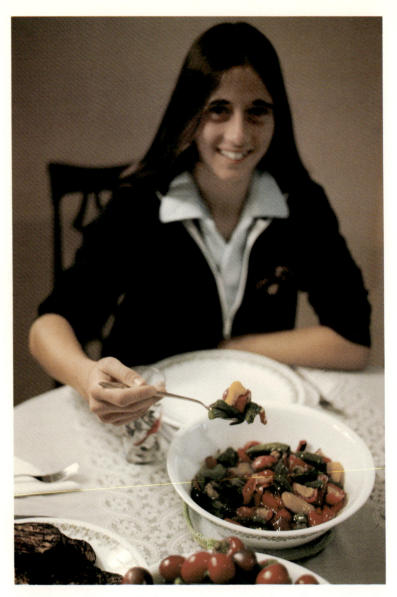

Our daughter, Dawn, reaches for a tempting spoonful of mixed red and green hot peppers that have been cooked in olive oil. In the foreground are charcoal broiled eggplant slices. During the summer, I place the peppers in foil with olive oil and crushed garlic cloves, turn up the foil edges and set the bagged foil package right on the barbeque grill. I cut the eggplant into thick slices, dip it in olive oil/ crushed garlic combination, sprinkle vegetable seasoning, and cook right on the barbeque grill. Can also be baked in an oven.

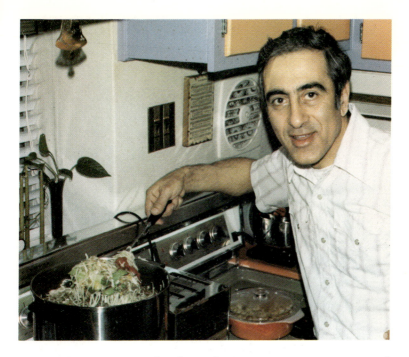

During the winter months the author prepares a 20-quart pot of cabbage soup at regular intervals. It is both a robust and very nutritious picker-upper that gives sustenance through the cold wintry days.

KIRBAN'S CABBAGE SOUP 10 Servings

In heavy bottom soup pot, combine:
- 2 lbs. beef small cubed
- 2 onions diced
- 6 carrots sliced
- 1 can (16 oz.) tomatoes
- 2 soup bones cracked
- 3 quarts water

Bring to boil; then simmer for 1 hour. Skim fat from top.

Then add:
- 3 lbs. cabbage diced
- 1 bay leaf
- 1½ teaspoons thyme
- ⅛ teaspoon cayenne pepper

Simmer an additional 45 minutes. Just before end of cooking period, add:
- ½ cup cider vinegar
- ¼ cup brown sugar (or ⅛ cup honey)

You will find this a very hearty and satisfying soup. For my own family, I multiply this recipe by 4 and make a large 20-quart pot of cabbage soup. It lasts us an entire week. If one has a cold or a stuffed nose this soup has a way of clearing the nasal passages. You will find Kirban's Cabbage Soup very robust and nutritious and a popular family meal. Be inventive. You can substitute lamb for beef. You can throw in a package of mixed frozen vegetables. You can leave out the meat and add some soup stock.

SALEM'S SALAD

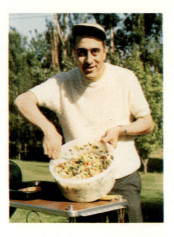

My parents were born in Lebanon. Their parents and grandparents showed them how to live off the bountiful, nutritious harvest from the land. The people in Lebanon thrive on burghul (bulgur). Bulgur is a cracked whole-grain wheat. They also eat in abundance eggplant, tomatoes, parsley, grapeleaves. They garnish their salads liberally with garlic, olive oil and lemon juice. The fresh lemon is as popular to the Lebanese as hamburgers are to the American!

Most of my young life was spent above Scranton in the small but beautiful towns of Clarks Summit, Tunkhannock and Schultzville. Here my mother passed down the traditions of the family and showed me how to make **Tabbouleh,** the salad par excellence! I make it 3 or 4 times every summer and everytime I make it differently. It is a salad in which you can use your creative ingenuity. It is highly nutritious. Make enough for an entire week. As it ages each day in the refrigerator the flavor seems to improve. But how can you improve on excellence!

Soak for 1 hour before preparing: **Serves 6**
    1 cup <u>fine</u> bulgur wheat*

It will greatly expand. Drain and squeeze out remaining water with your hands. In a large salad bowl, place the dried bulgur with:
- **4 finely chopped scallions**
- **1 onion diced**

Squeeze ingredients with your hand so that the juice of onions penetrates the bulgur. Season to taste with vegetable seasonings. Then add:
- **1 cup parsley finely chopped**
- **2½ tablespoons dried mint**
  (or 4 tablespoons fresh mint chopped)
- **4 large tomatoes diced**
- **½ cup olive oil**
- **Juice of 4 lemons**

Mix well. For greater exhilaration, I place **two chopped garlic cloves** in a cup with **3 tablespoons of olive oil.** I crush the garlic with a pestle (or spoon) so that the aroma of the garlic becomes an integral part of the oil. I then place this "golden glow" into the salad mix. With that addition the salad will become the pièce de résistance (the principal dish of the meal)! Or, as Aunt Effie would say: *"Not only will it lower your blood pressure but it will keep your enemies away from you."* To which I might add: *"And your friends, also!"*

* Bulgur wheat can be purchased at your local health food store. Make sure it is the fine (not coarse) grain. Also be sure it is plain bulgur wheat, not flavored or spiced.

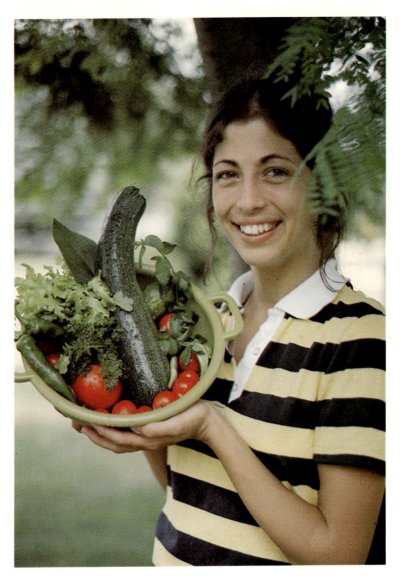

Our daughter, Doreen, with a bountiful harvest of vegetables just picked from our backyard garden. How many items can you see? She is holding zucchini squash, comfrey, lettuce, peppers, cherry and regular tomatoes, cucumbers, mint, parsley and string beans (10 items). We also grew watermelon, okra, celery, carrots and beets. We prepared the soil according to Dr. Carey Reams' recommendations and the results were fantastic!

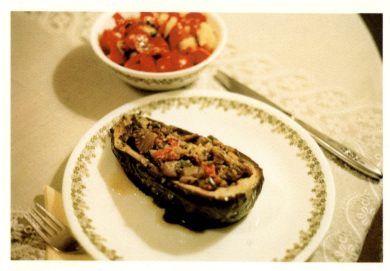

Stuffed eggplant makes a most appetizing dish the entire family will enjoy. Include a sparkling garden salad with tomatoes, cucumbers, parsley, chopped onions and mint. Use any salad dressing but why not try olive oil. And liberally squeeze fresh lemon juice on your salad!

ESTHER'S STUFFED EGGPLANT   **6 Servings**

Preheat oven to 350°.
Bring a large pot of water to a boil and add:
    3 eggplants medium
Cover and simmer for 5 to 10 minutes. Drain and cool under running water. Cut in half <u>lengthwise</u> and carefully scoop out the pulp with a spoon or grapefruit knife, leaving a 1/2" thick shell. Chop the pulp and set aside.

Heat in your largest skillet:
    ½ cup olive oil
and sauté until transparent:
    1½ cups onion chopped
    2 cloves garlic minced
Add:
      eggplant pulp
    1 1-lb. can tomatoes drained
    1 lb. ground lamb (optional)
Cook over low heat stirring occasionally for 15 minutes. Season with vegetable seasonings to taste.
Add:
      breadcrumbs
      parsley
      mint
Fill eggplant shells with mixture. Arrange eggplant halves in an oiled baking pan. Drizzle a little olive oil over each eggplant. If desired, sprinkle Parmesan cheese on top. Bake for 30 minutes in 350° oven.

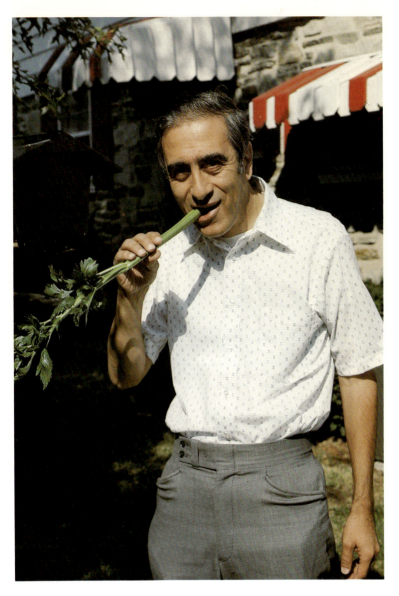

Learn the secret of relaxing. When you feel a headache coming on . . . when the events of the day have made you tense . . . or you're a bundle of nerves . . . take a break from your activities, take a tip from the Author. Go outside, bask in the sun and chew on a stalk or two of celery! Take a celery-break instead of a candy or cookie or coffee break! You'll notice the refreshing difference immediately.

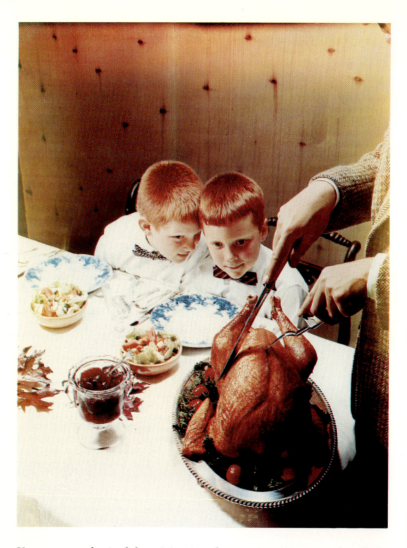

You can see the joyful anticipation these twins convey as they look forward to a tantalizing turkey dinner. Train your children even at one-year-old to develop a liking for wholesome foods. If you start feeding them candy, cookies and cakes you are training them to develop bad eating habits that will reflect in their health problems in future years. Many will become hyperactive. Many will not be able to cope with problems in later life. Next time, give them a carrot stick instead of candy; a celery stalk instead of cake; a pear instead of a popsicle. Go easy on meat and stress raw vegetables and fruits.

DINAH
The woman who went sightseeing

Name Means: Justice
Identification: Daughter of Jacob and Leah.
Scripture Reference: Genesis 34

Dinah was young and daring and loved to sightsee.

One day she stole away from the tents of her father to see how the other part of the world was living. She was awed by the oriental trappings of nearby Shechem (now Nablus) in Israel. While sightseeing Prince Shechem seduced her and she went to his palace. Had Dinah stayed at home she could have averted a terrible massacre. Her wandering brought about disaster.

The young prince offered to marry Dinah and to pay her father Jacob, a sum of money according to Hebrew law (Deuteronomy 22:28,29). At first it appeared that such an arrangement could be worked out. But the sons of Jacob, although seeming to agree, sought revenge and slew all the males in the city of Shechem including the young prince. The tragedy caused Jacob to reconsecrate his life and he made an altar at Bethel to God.

Nothing more is said about Dinah. Perhaps she learned a bitter lesson and spent the rest of her life trying to please her family through dedicated service.

DINAH'S DATE BARS
16 Bars

Preheat oven to 325°.
Oil bottom of an 8 x 8-inch pan.
Sift together:

- 1/2 cup brown rice flour
- 1/2 cup oat flour

Set above aside and combine:
- 3/4 cup nuts chopped
- 1 cup dates chopped
- 1/4 cup wheat germ

In medium bowl, combine:
- 1/2 cup sifted carob powder
- 1/2 cup oil
- 1/3 cup honey
- 2 eggs beaten

Add:
- sifted flour
- date mixture
- 1 teaspoon vanilla extract

Pour batter into pan. Bake in oven for 25 minutes. Cut into bars.

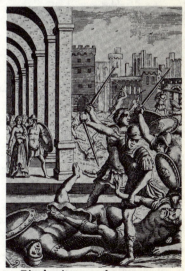

Dinah witnesses the massacre.

CAROB CHIP COOKIES
Yield: 36 cookies

Preheat oven to 350°.
In a large mixing bowl, cream:
- 1/2 cup butter, softened
- 1 cup honey

Then add:
- 2 eggs slightly beaten

Add:
- 2¼ cups whole wheat flour
- 2 teaspoons baking powder
- 1 cup nuts chopped
- 1 teaspoon vanilla
- 1 package carob chips

Mix well. Then chill dough in refrigerator for one hour. Drop by the teaspoonful on oiled cookie sheet. Bake in oven at 350° until lightly browned (about 10-12 minutes). (Carob chips can be secured from your local health food store.) (Basic recipe from *The Forget-About-Meat Cookbook* by Karen Brooks, published by Rodale Press, 1974.)

RAISIN MOLASSES BARS
About 30 2 x 2½-inch Bars

Preheat oven to 375°.
Melt:
- 6 tablespoons butter

When cooled slightly, stir in:
- 1/4 cup honey
- 2/3 cup dark molasses
- 1 slightly beaten egg
- 1 teaspoon vanilla

Sift together:
- 1 cup unbleached white flour with wheat germ
- 1/8 teaspoon baking soda
- 1 teaspoon cinnamon
- 1/8 teaspoon cloves
- 1/8 teaspoon ginger

Add to the flour:
- 1 cup raisins
- 1/2 cup chopped nuts

Blend together all ingredients. Pour into a greased 10½ x 15½-inch cookie sheet. Bake about 12 minutes. When cool, cut into 2 x 2½-inch bars. For the adventurer, brush top with fresh lemon juice and sprinkle on cinnamon.

REAMS' REVIEW SOUP

Reams' Review Soup is sometimes known as Salvation Soup (all the saved left-overs). Here's a chance to exercise all your ingenuity. Even a man can make this soup. When vegetables are added to soups, most people sauteé them first in oil. They find this helps to seal in the flavor of the vegetables. It also keeps them firm when they are added to the soup. The secret of a good soup lies in its "stock" or base. Below is a suggested beef stock recipe.

BEEF SOUP Stock
Yield: 6 cups

Soup stock should be made at least one day before you plan to use it.

Brown in heavy bottom 4-quart soup pot:
- 1 cracked beef shin bone

Then add:
- 2 stalks celery with leaves, chopped
- 2 carrots, chopped
- 2 onions, diced

Add:
- 2 quarts cold water
- sea salt to taste
- parsley sprigs
- 1 cup tomatoes

Simmer for 3 hours on low heat. If vinegar is added to the stock while simmering, it will dissolve the calcium in the bones and these nutrients will become a part of the stock. The vinegar smell and taste cook away as the stock simmers.

Discard bones and vegetables. You may wish to remove the marrow from the bones and stir it in the broth. Strain the stock, cool the remaining broth and refrigerate. Before using this stock, be sure to remove the fat from the top and discard it.

WEEK 1

Dr. Reams:
What foods cause worms?

Worms are caused because the gastric juices are too dilute. The gastric juices are too dilute because of a lack of calcium in your diet and a lack of oxygen. Your energy level is too low. Whenever the gastric juices are strong enough it does away with the worms. You can get them from simply shaking hands from a friend who has a pet or petting a pet or walking barefoot.

* * *

Dr. Reams:
Is popcorn ok to eat?

Yes, about a teacup full a year!

* * *

Dr. Reams:
Should liquids be taken at a meal?

It is best to drink liquids between meals. Of course you will have to drink a little liquid to take your minerals with your meals. But other liquids should not be taken until 20-30 minutes after your main course.

> Note: Although Sunday is the first day of the week . . . in this book . . . for the convenience of modern diet purposes, we have begun each week with Monday.

> Bless the Lord, O my soul, and forget not all His benefits: Who forgiveth all thine iniquities; Who healeth all thy diseases . . . *Psalm 103:1-3*

WEEK 1 DAY 1
MONDAY

QUESTIONS FREQUENTLY ASKED . . .

Why Breakfast, Dinner, Supper? Shouldn't the big meal be at night?

Most people have been conditioned to Breakfast, Lunch and Dinner . . . eating their biggest meal in the evening. This is wrong! A large meal eaten in the evening just opens the door for a host of illnesses in later life.

Lunchtime should be <u>DINNER</u>, where a substantial meal is eaten. At this time, you still have a few hours to work it off and utilize the energy. But if you eat a large meal in the evening, what do you do? You relax, then go to bed. And problems occur.

You will find this **7 Week Diet Plan** a Breakfast—Dinner—Supper plan with hearty meals designed for breakfast and midday. That's why we call it Breakfast, **Dinner** and Supper.

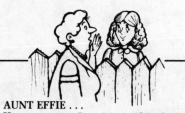

AUNT EFFIE . . .
Have you seen Cora Mae's Shingles?
No, but the rest of her house is a mess! Oughta have her body chemistry checked, first-off. I tried a "triple-header" when I had them. First, took daily a vitamin-mineral supplement. Then, rubbed Vitamin E oil on the Shingles. And then alternated with Lemon water applied liberally. It worked!

BREAKFAST
1 fruit   1/2 grapefruit
1 toast   butter
Hot shredded wheat cooked in skim milk
Milk (6 ounces)
Hot herb tea or coffee

DINNER
Fresh vegetable salad
Cornbread
Cup of vegetable broth
Abishag's Casserole *

SUPPER
Leafy vegetable salad
1 slice of whole wheat toast
Jacob's Birthright Soup *
1 yogurt
Hot herb tea or skim milk

* **See index for recipe.**

LOOKING AHEAD
Tuesday
Soak grits overnight tonight. Buy vegetarian breakfast sausage and chicken, asparagus, corn, squash, graham crackers, apple juice.
Wednesday
Buy oranges, oatmeal, salad items, chow mein, rice, cranberry juice, yogurt, bananas, meatless Irish stew, and molasses cookies.

> Is anything too hard for the Lord?
> Genesis 18:14

WEEK 1 DAY 2
TUESDAY

QUESTIONS FREQUENTLY ASKED . . .

What is the first number in the Reams Equation?

The first number in the Reams Urine/Saliva equation is Sugar. The normal sugar level is 1.5. If this number is in the 6.0 range, Dr. Reams states that it indicates that the individual is a borderline diabetic.

This is a combined sugar reading read by a refractometer. Urine sugars are measured as opposed to blood sugars because blood sugars tend to elevate or depress several times within an hour. Dr. Reams believes the urine sugar reading provides a more accurate reading.

Those with a sugar reading of 5.5 or above should **not** drink the Lemon water combination. Instead they should drink only distilled water. The reason: Lemon water would release the toxins too quickly in your body and could drive up your salts and urea to an unacceptable level.

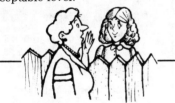

AUNT EFFIE . . .
My child coughs a spell some nights.

Old Angus, he was a hard one for me to raise. Some nights he'd cough so loud he broke the sound barrier. I wrestled up some Comfrey tea . . . about 1/2 cup . . . let it steep good and added a teaspoon of honey. Angus went back to sleep within 15 minutes. He slept all night!

BREAKFAST

1 fruit	apple
1 toast	butter

Grits
    Soak overnight and cook slowly for about two hours until creamy — add 1 can of whole kernal corn that has been through the blender (one can of corn to about 15 servings)
Serve with 2 links vegetarian sausage
Hot herb tea or coffee

DINNER

Fresh vegetable salad
Corn bread
Asparagus on toast with brown gravy
Steamed squash
2 slices (very thin) vegetarian chicken
Green drink *

SUPPER

Fresh vegetable salad
1 slice whole wheat toast
Reams' Review Soup *
Peach (1/2) on Graham cracker
Apple juice (4 ounces)
Cup of herb tea

* See index for recipe.

LOOKING AHEAD

Wednesday
Oranges, oatmeal, salad items, chow mein, rice, cranberry juice, yogurt, bananas, meatless Irish stew, and molasses cookies.

Thursday
Eggs, onions, vegetarian bacon, hamburger, turnip greens, apricot halves.

> And, behold, a woman, which was diseased with an issue of blood twelve years . . . touched the hem of His garment . . . And when Jesus saw her, He said, Daughter, be of good comfort; thy faith hath made thee whole. . . .
> Matthew 9:20, 22

WEEK 1 DAY 3
WEDNESDAY

What is the second number in the Reams Equation?

The second number registers the pH level. Dr. Reams states that the normal pH for urine and saliva is 6.40. If the level drops below 6.40 the body cannot utilize Vitamin C. He believes it is important that one's body be brought to the normal pH so there is no energy loss. Continued energy loss initially evidences itself by fatigue.

A drop in pH would be an increase in acidity. A rise in pH would be an increase in alkalinity. The top figure is the urine pH reading; the bottom figure is the saliva pH reading.

The saliva pH gives an indication of the bile strength and also gives an indication as to which direction the numbers are going. Dr. Reams believes it important that one's body be brought back to the normal pH so there is no energy loss. Continued energy loss eventually ends in major illness.

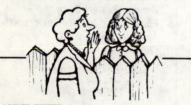

AUNT EFFIE . . .
What can Penelope do for Eczema?

The old-fashioned housewife's menus were carefully thought out. The modern housewife's are carefully thawed out. Penelope ought to eat right . . . first. My Aunt Bertha had the same problem. She'd take two teaspoons of blackstrap molasses in a glass of skim milk twice daily.

BREAKFAST
1 fruit — orange
1 toast — butter
Oatmeal with raisins
  honey & allspice added to taste
Milk (6 ounces)
Herb tea or coffee

DINNER
Fresh vegetable salad
Corn muffin
Chicken Chow Mein on rice
Green beans
Boiled onion
1 yogurt
Cranberry juice (4 ounces)

SUPPER
Salad - leafy vegetable
1 banana
Eve's Meatless Stew *
Apple juice
Corn chips **
1 slice whole wheat toast
Herb tea

* See index for recipe.

** Health Valley or Dr. Bronner brand or similar. Check with your health food store.

LOOKING AHEAD
Thursday
Eggs, onions, vegetarian bacon, hamburger, turnip greens, apricot halves.

Friday
Grapefruit, millet, allspice, green beans, peppers for stuffing, beets, vegetarian chili, corn crisps, yogurt.

> And Jesus went about all the cities and villages, teaching in their synagogues, and preaching the Gospel of the kingdom, and healing every sickness and every disease among the people.... *Matthew 9:35*

WEEK 1 DAY 4
THURSDAY

What is the third number in the Reams Equation?

The third number in the Reams Equation registers the salt level. Dr. Reams states that the normal salt level is 6C to 7C. Too much salt is the cause of many heart conditions. When the salt reading is 20 and above, Dr. Reams believes the diet should be corrected quickly. The salt reading indicates the combined tissue salts being thrown off by the body through the urine. A high salt reading would indicate a high level of tissue salt retention. However, one cannot look at the individual numbers. The overall pattern of numbers have to be analyzed.

When one's salt level is high, the heart is working too hard and often you can hear your heart beat. Dr. Reams believes the distilled water and lemon water program is beneficial to reducing the salt level towards the normal level.

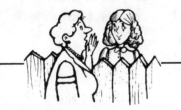

AUNT EFFIE...
How can I help digestion?
Most people think parsley is the food you push aside to see what is under it. You're supposed to eat that green stuff! It's good for digestion and is loaded with Vitamin C. And I've heard Doc Reams recommend 2 teaspoons of Heinz Sweet Pickle vinegar for each meal.

BREAKFAST
1 fruit — banana
1 toast — butter
Wilderness Wok *
2 Stripples
  (vegetarian bacon)
Herb tea or coffee

DINNER
Fresh vegetable salad
Corn bread
English hamburger gravy on toast
  Soak blood from raw hamburger. Cook fry in skillet until done. Put into larger pot. Add cold water and bring to boil. Brown gluten flour and add to boiling meat.
  Add can cream and spices
Steamed carrot
Turnip greens

SUPPER
Fresh leafy green vegetable salad
1 slice whole wheat toast
Vashti's Vegetable Soup *
Yogurt
Glass of skim milk (6 ounces)
Apricot halves (2) on Graham cracker
Herb tea

* See index for recipe.

LOOKING AHEAD
Friday
Grapefruit, millet, allspice, green beans, peppers for stuffing, beets, vegetarian chili, corn crisps, yogurt.

Saturday
Oranges, apples, carrots, parsnips, pineapple slices, cranberry juice, whole wheat bread, grape juice.

> Confess your faults one to another, and pray one for another, that ye may be healed. The effectual fervent prayer of a righteous man availeth much. *James 5:16*

WEEK 1   DAY 5

FRIDAY

What is the fourth number in the Reams Equation?

The fourth number in the Reams Equation registers the Albumin. The normal level is .04M. The Albumin count is the number of minute particles in the urine. Dr. Reams believes that urine in a healthy individual (with certain exceptions) should be clear (transparent).

One with a perfect number of .04M would be throwing off very little cellular debris. However, when the number starts to rise, your body is breaking down faster than it is building up. You begin to lose reserve energy.

Normal Albumin is .04M or 40,000 particles per liter. Many people have an Albumin reading of 4M. This means 4,000,000 particles per liter. This would mean your body is throwing out **100** times the amount of cellular debris it should normally! One with perfect numbers would be throwing off very little cellular debris.

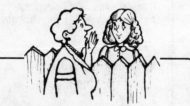

AUNT EFFIE...
What can I do for hay fever?

Honey, my grandfather suffered from hay fever so bad his nose ran like Niagara Falls. His daddy went out and got him some Comfrey planted ... that's the funny plant with the furry leaves. Granddaddy would fold the leaves with the fur inside and chew two 6-inch leaves a day!

BREAKFAST

1 fruit   1/2 grapefruit
1 toast   butter
Ezekiel's Ecstasy (Millet) *
Herb tea or coffee

DINNER

Fresh vegetable salad
Corn bread
Solomon's Celery Soup *
Corn chips served with soup
Green beans - steamed
Stuffed pepper - use vegetables instead of meat for stuffing
Small whole beets (3)

SUPPER

Fresh green leafy salad
1 slice whole wheat toast
1 vegetarian chili
Corn chips
1 yogurt
Herb tea

* **See index for recipe.**

> Soak granola overnight in skim milk in refrigerator for tomorrow's breakfast.

LOOKING AHEAD

Saturday
Oranges, apples, carrots, parsnips, pineapple slices, cranberry juice, whole wheat bread, grape juice.
Sunday
Bananas, okra, vegetarian chicken, ears of corn, eggplant, mushrooms, apple juice and Jello.

> He healeth the broken in heart, and bindeth up their wounds ... Great is our Lord, and of great power; His understanding is infinite.
> *Psalm 147:3, 5*

WEEK 1 DAY 6
SATURDAY

What is the fifth number in the Reams Equation?

The fifth number in the Reams Equation is the Urea. The normal urea level is 3 over 3, or a total of 6. The top reading is the urine cationic nitrate nitrogen reading. The bottom reading is the saliva anionic ammoniacal nitrogen reading. Dr. Reams believes if the total of these reaches 20, the heart is overworking and fatigue is evidenced. This part of the Equation measures the level of undigested proteins in the body chemistry.

When protein disgestion is slow or not normal, excess protein remains in the bowels. In the colon these improperly digested proteins ferment, putrify and produce toxins. These toxins are absorbed and enter the blood and lymph systems. They change the relative acidity of the body tissues and interfere with proper metabolism and tissue oxygenation.

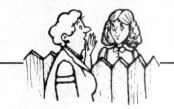

AUNT EFFIE ...
Why so hung up on Lemon Water?
Honey, if life hands you a lemon, don't sour up your face. Turn it into lemonade and share your blessings. Doc Reams and Lemon Water is a dynamic duo. Anytime I've got an itch that persists, SPLASH goes the Lemon Water. Anytime I got something I don't want ... SPLASH goes the Lemon Water.

BREAKFAST
1 fruit — orange
1 toast — butter
Granola
Baked apple
Herb tea or coffee

DINNER
Fresh vegetable salad
Corn bread
Anna's Steamed Delight *
Cranberry juice (6 ounces)
Raisin molasses bars *
1 slice of pineapple on Graham cracker with one marshmallow

SUPPER
Fresh green leafy salad
1 slice whole wheat toast
Caleb's carrot soup *
1 yogurt
Grape juice (6 ounces)
Herb tea

* See index for recipe.

> (Soak whole wheat berries tonight for Monday's breakfast.)

LOOKING AHEAD
Sunday
Bananas, okra, vegetarian chicken, corn on the cob, eggplant, mushrooms, apple juice and Jello.
Monday
Apples, whole wheat berries, yellow squash, spinach, eggs, carrots, vegetarian turkey, cauliflower, fresh tomatoes.

> They that wait upon the Lord shall renew their strength; they shall mount up with wings as eagles; they shall run, and not be weary; and they shall walk and not faint. *Isaiah 40:31*

WEEK 1 DAY 7
SUNDAY

What is the purpose of using fresh lemon juice?

Fresh (not reconstituted) lemon juice acts as an anionic substance. Anions interacting with cations produce energy. Outside of the lemon . . . all other foods are cationic. The liver requires energy in large quantities in order to maintain its enzyme systems, bile production, its role as body detoxifyer as well as other functions which utilize a vast quantity of enzymes. When one's body does not have sufficient anionic substances, the energy level drops because we are not assimilating our food properly. With the majority of our food being cationic in nature, one can easily see the need for the lemon juice to provide the anionic requirements.

Must I take lemon water all my life?

Those who take lemon water will find that when one's body chemistry comes to the normal or near normal equation the lemon water can be stopped.

AUNT EFFIE . . .
How can I avoid additives?

Listen, child . . . if you tickle the earth with a hoe, she laughs with a harvest. Trouble is food manufacturers want to help Mother Nature and Father Money. They add over 1100 flavoring additives and a host of preservatives. Start farming and stop buying.

BREAKFAST
1 fruit — banana
1 toast — butter
All juice breakfast: (choice of)
  carrot juice (6 ounces)
  cranberry juice (6 ounces)
  grape juice (6 ounces)
  skim milk (6 ounces)
Herb tea or coffee

DINNER
Fresh vegetable salad
Whole wheat (homemade) bread
Steamed or fried okra
Green beans
Desert Jello
2 slices of vegetarian chicken
1 ear of corn
carrot juice (6 ounces)

SUPPER
Fresh green leafy salad
1 slice toast
Vashti's vegetable soup *
Eggplant with mushroom
Jello
  (Chop celery and banana; add to grape juice with Knox gelatin. Shredded coconut on top.)
Apple juice (4 ounces)

* See index for recipe

(Slow cook whole wheat berries today for Monday's breakfast.)

LOOKING AHEAD
Monday
Apples, whole wheat berries, yellow squash, spinach, eggs, carrots, vegetarian turkey, cauliflower, fresh tomatoes.

Tuesday
Cream of Wheat, halved peaches, graham crackers, vegetable scallops, Rye crisp, raisins and coconut.

WEEK 2

Dr. Reams:
What is wrong with tuna fish and bonita?

Both are skin fish and they digest too quickly in your body, the same as shellfish, catfish and pork. They digest in a period of about 3 hours. It should take 18 hours.

* * *

Dr. Reams:
Do sweet potatoes turn into alcohol in the body and are they a good food?

I have never seen a case where sweet potatoes turn into alcohol but I have seen this happen in white potatoes. This is one reason why we recommend that white potatoes be eaten infrequently.

* * *

Dr. Reams:
Are one day fasts helpful in cleaning out the body?

One day fasts are excellent for cleaning out the body providing you don't go back to eating the wrong kinds of food.

* * *

Dr. Reams:
Should children eat meats?

No! Children under 12 should not eat meats. Instead give them soybean vegetarian meats to meet their protein requirements.

43

> Although Moses was one hundred and twenty years old when he died, his eye was not dim, nor his vigor abated. *Deuteronomy 34:7*

WEEK 2   DAY 1
MONDAY

How do you define illness?

Dr. Carey Reams defines illness as due to loss of energy resulting in lowered resistance. He believes that a person starts on the road to illness the first day his body burns up more energy than he is able to assimilate from his foods.

The urine/saliva test determines the energy equation. Dr. Reams believes if a person gets well, it is because his body chemistry has changed closer to the biological norm. This increases the body's energy reserves and allows the body to heal itself.

God has created for you a well-functioning body at birth (unless you were born with birth defects). He entrusted this body to you. If you find yourself ill, it could be because your improper diet over the years has taken its toll. The wrong foods rob you of energy and toxins begin to build up in your system. It's time to change your diet!

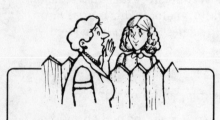

AUNT EFFIE ...
My hubby's got ulcers.

Being a woman is a terribly difficult trade, since it consists principally of dealing with men. If hubby has stomach ulcers ... the lemon is not his friend. But cabbage is. Try giving him some cabbage juice a little at a time each day ... till he gets used to it. And don't nag!

BREAKFAST

1 fruit   apple
1 toast   butter
Whole wheat berries
   (Soaked for 24 hours; then cooked slowly for 4 to 6 hours.)
Skim milk
Herb tea or coffee

DINNER

Fresh vegetable salad
Corn bread
Yellow squash
Spinach with boiled egg
Steamed carrot (whole)
2 slices of vegetarian turkey
Deborah's Delight *

SUPPER

Fresh green leafy salad
1 slice of toast
Creamed cauliflower
Solomon's celery soup *
Fresh tomato (2 slices)
1 yogurt
Cranberry juice (4 ounces)

* See index for recipe.

LOOKING AHEAD

Tuesday
Cream of Wheat, halved peaches, graham crackers, vegetable scallops, Rye crisp, raisins and coconut.

Wednesday
Vegetarian bacon, rice, eggs, onions, halved pears, pumpernickel bread, asparagus, corn on the cob, banana pudding.

> Like snow in summer and like rain in harvest, so honor is not fitting for a fool ... Like a sparrow in its wandering, as the swallow in her flying, So a curse without a cause does not come. *Proverbs 26:1, 2*

WEEK 2   DAY 2

TUESDAY

What does Dr. Reams mean by "cause and effect?"

For every cause there is a reaction or an effect. Dr. Reams believes one should go direct to the **cause** of illness and not treat initially the **effect**. Most drugs treat the **effect**. If you have a cold, you may be given an antibiotic which may temporarily help in the treatment of the **effect**; that is, stuffy nose, headache, etc. But the cold is an indication that your body chemistry is not in line and your reserve energy level is dropping. Getting at the **cause** of illness is important.

Some people who are nervous or high strung take Valium. This tranquilizer has a calmative, soothing **effect** but it does not treat the **cause**!

Cause is the loss of the perfect chemistry of one's body. The **effect** of this loss is illness. Dr. Reams believes one will never regain perfect health by treating **effects**. One must go to the **cause**.

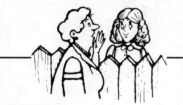

AUNT EFFIE ...
I've got "dishpan hands."

3 tablespoons of whole or cracked flaxseed overnight in a pint of warm water. In the morning, boil mixture, then strain to remove the jell, discard seeds, add a pint of **clear** vinegar. Then add 3 ounces of glycerin. Boil again. Then beat with eggbeater for 1 minute. Bottle. Dampen hands with mixture and rub in.

BREAKFAST

1 fruit	banana
1 toast	butter

Cream of wheat
Boiled egg
Vegetarian sausage (2 thin slices)
Peach (1/2) on Graham cracker
Herb tea or coffee

DINNER

Fresh vegetable salad
Corn bread
Cup of vegetable broth
Dorcas's Dream casserole *
Dinah's Date Bar *

SUPPER

Fresh green leafy vegetable salad
1 slice toast
Tomato soup
Rye crisp
Fresh fruit Jello   pineapple
Apple & raisins soaked with coconut
Herb tea

* See index for recipe.

LOOKING AHEAD

Wednesday
Vegetarian bacon, rice, eggs, onions, halved pears, pumpernickel bread, asparagus, corn on the cob, banana pudding.

Thursday
Carrots, V-8 juice, salad items, corn, vegetarian corn beef, Mulligan stew, celery, fruit salad.

> And Asa in the thirty and ninth year of his reign was diseased in his feet, until his disease was exceeding great, yet in his disease, he sought not to the Lord, but to the physicians. And Asa slept with his fathers.... 2 Chronicles 16:12, 13

WEEK 2 DAY 3
WEDNESDAY

Should I start a fast or light diet immediately?

First check with your doctor. Those with high ureas or very high combined salt numbers may not tolerate an immediate fast or light diet.

What can I expect on a fast or light diet program?

Some have reported that they have broken out in hives. This is a sign that one's body chemistry is changing. Your body will go into a withdrawal pattern as it gets rid of excess sugar, drug residues, accumulated wastes and dead cellular debris. If you have been eating the wrong foods over the years you have accumulated a lot of waste in your body. And as your body starts to throw this off, you will have reactions. You may experience headaches, irritability and upset stomach. It is important to rest and maintain your fluid intake faithfully.

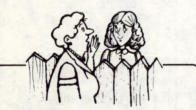

AUNT EFFIE...
Cora Mae's sinus is acting up

Cora Mae is full of troubles. Listen, you can't keep trouble from coming, but don't give it a chair to sit in! Hot peppers ought to clear her nose like an expressway. Angus used to eat hot peppers, take three 30 mg. zinc tablets a day and he reduced his meat intake. Man, Angus could eat!

BREAKFAST
1 fruit — orange
1 toast — butter
Wilderness Wok *
Stripples (vegetarian bacon)
Pear (1/2) on Graham cracker
Herb tea or coffee

DINNER
Fresh vegetable salad
Homemade pumpernickel bread
Green beans
Onion soup - 1 cup
Asparagus
Corn on the cob
Raisin molasses bars *
Hot herb tea (cold tea in summer)

SUPPER
Fresh green leafy salad
1 slice whole wheat toast
Reams' Review Soup *
Skim milk
Corn chips
Banana pudding
Herb tea

* See index for recipe.

LOOKING AHEAD
Thursday
Carrots, V-8 juice, salad items, corn, vegetarian corn beef, Mulligan stew, celery, fruit salad.
Friday
Melon, millet, eggs, vegetarian sausage, cabbage, zucchini squash, date nut bread, apple juice, orange juice.

> Be not among winebibbers; among riotous eaters of flesh: for the drunkard and glutton shall come to poverty. Hell and destruction are never full; so the eyes of man are never satisfied. Proverbs 23:20, 21; 27:20

WEEK 2 DAY 4
THURSDAY

Why are raw foods recommended?

Remember this. Live foods for live bodies! Raw foods are alive. They still have active enzymes. And when they are digested in your body, they can quickly offer life energy to your body. Another bonus . . . they are a natural source of roughage and cellulose. Raw foods not only regulate the rate at which that which you have eaten is propelled through your colon, but they also act as a brush removing the encrustations on the colon wall.

Cellulose has another advantage. It is an excellent natural detoxifier. It attracts certain toxic substances in the colon so they can't be absorbed into your system.

One may wonder then . . . why not eat everything raw? Eating raw food exclusively would detoxify you too fast. Then, too, your bile in your liver may be too weak to aid the digestion of raw foods properly.

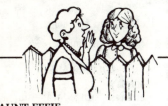

AUNT EFFIE . . .
Fergus is 25 and still has Acne!
Well, Fergus is committing suicide with a fork . . . eating so much pork, fried foods and cakes, candy and pastries. First, get his colon moving daily. His colon is so clogged up it must be run by the Government. Give him bran. Give him a zinc supplement. Splash on Lemon Water daily. Eat right.

BREAKFAST
1 fruit — pear
1 toast — butter
Shredded carrot salad
   with raisins, coconut, Jello
2 Graham crackers
V-8 juice (4 ounces)
Herb tea or coffee

DINNER
Fresh vegetable salad
Corn bread
Elizabeth's casserole *
2 slices vegetarian beef
Delilah's milk shake
   Banana shake
      Concoct a milk shake with sliced bananas in blender
Hot or cold herb tea

SUPPER
Fresh leafy green salad
1 slice whole wheat toast
Kirban's Cabbage soup *
Celery juice (4 ounces)
Mixed fruit salad (1/2) cup served on Graham crackers
Herb tea

* See index for recipe.

LOOKING AHEAD
Friday
Melon, millet, eggs, vegetarian sausage, cabbage, zucchini squash, date nut bread, apple juice, orange juice.
Saturday
Bananas, grits, grape juice, Hush puppies, baked beans, corn on the cob, yogurt, celery, vegetarian vegetable soup, Boston bread.

> Fret not thyself because of evildoers, neither be thou envious against the workers of iniquity. For they shall soon be cut down like the grass, and wither as the green herb. *Psalm 37:1-2*

WEEK 2　　DAY 5

FRIDAY

How can I avoid foods with additives?

Admittedly, it is next to impossible. The use of additives has **doubled** in the past 15 years, from 400 million pounds to more than 800 million pounds. Today, over 3000 chemicals are deliberately added to our foods. The average American consumes 4 pounds of chemical preservatives, stabilizers, colorings, flavorings and other additives each year! It is difficult to avoid eating some additives.

Where possible, grow your own food and freeze food for winter months. Buy your foods from reliable health food stores or vegetable truck farms you have confidence in.

Buy your grains from your local health food store and grind them or ask them to grind them for you. Store in glass containers with tight lids.

A healthy, nutritional program will help flush out additives from your system.

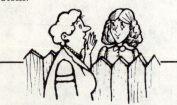

AUNT EFFIE . . .
Penelope is so depressed!
Penelope should learn that happiness is like a potato salad. Share it and you have a picnic. Penelope should stop feeling sorry for herself, find her faith in God, feed and water her body properly. It is God's Temple. The Sermon on the Mount can lift us out of the Valley of Depression.

BREAKFAST
1 fruit　　　　　　melon in season
1 toast　　　　　　　　　　butter
Ezekiel's Ecstasy (Millet) *
Scrambled eggs
Vegetarian sausage
V-8 juice (4 ounces)
Herb tea or coffee

DINNER
Fresh vegetable salad
Corn bread muffins
Corned beef and cabbage
Zucchini squash
Green drink *
Steamed carrot
Date nut bread (1 thin slice)
Peach (1/2)
Hot or cold herb tea

SUPPER
Fresh green leafy salad
1 slice of whole wheat toast
Celery soup
Corn chips
Apple juice (6 ounces)
Orange juice (6 ounces)
Hot herb tea

* **See index for recipe.**

　Soak grits tonight.

LOOKING AHEAD
Saturday
Bananas, grits, grape juice, Hush puppies, baked beans, corn on the cob, yogurt, celery, vegetarian vegetable soup, Boston Bread
Sunday
Grapefruit, Herb tea, apple butter, graham crackers, cottage cheese, peas, vegetarian chicken, sweet potatoes, asparagus soup.

> And God said, Behold, I have given you every herb bearing seed, which is upon the face of all the earth, and every tree, in the which is the fruit of a tree yielding seed; to you it shall be for meat. *Genesis 1:29*

WEEK 2 DAY 6
SATURDAY

Should I drink coffee or tea?

Don't drink commercial teas. They are poison to the liver. Herb teas, however, are very beneficial.

One cup of coffee or tea contains about 90mg. of caffeine. But commercial teas also contain tannin, or tannic acid, which is considered harmful. The English people drink multiple cups of tea daily. That's why they have bags under their eyes. One can usually spot an excessive tea drinker. He or she has bags under their eyes. Check out your friends and see if this isn't true!

It is better not to drink coffee nor commercial tea. The lesser of the two evils is coffee. And, if you drink coffee, don't drink decaffinated coffee . . . says Dr. Reams. Decaffinated coffee is loaded with chemical preservatives. Better to drink freshly perked coffee. If you are a heavy coffee or tea drinker, don't stop abruptly. Taper off slowly over a period of one month.

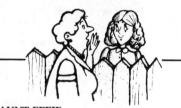

AUNT EFFIE . . .
Penelope has "hot flashes."

Penelope, honey, couldn't find joy in an ice cream cone. She'd claim the ice cream was too cold! Her hot flashes are from giving her husband a cold shoulder. What she needs is Vitamin E and a good mineral supplement with calciums. And have her body chemistry read!

BREAKFAST
1 fruit — banana
1 toast — butter
Granny's Grits.
   Serve with raisins added as a cereal. See page 37 for recipe.
Grape juice (6 ounces)
Herb tea or coffee

DINNER
Fresh vegetable salad
Hush puppies
Fish with tarter sauce and lemon (Any scaled fish)
Baked beans
Corn on the cob
Yogurt
Raisin molasses bars *
1 stalk of celery

SUPPER
Fresh leafy green salad
1 slice toast — butter
Vashti's vegetable soup *
Corn chips
V-8 juice (6 ounces)
Boston brown bread with peach half
Herb tea

* See index for recipe.

LOOKING AHEAD
Sunday
Grapefruit, Herb tea, apple butter, graham crackers, cottage cheese, peas, vegetarian chicken, sweet potatoes, asparagus soup.
Monday
Granola, corn bread, sauerkraut, vegetarian hot dogs, carrots, corn cake, orange juice, raisin pie, corn chips, green pea and celery soup.

> Trust in the Lord, and do good; so shalt thou dwell in the land, and verily thou shalt be fed. Delight thyself also in the Lord; and He shall give thee the desires of thine heart. *Psalm 37:3-4*

WEEK 2   DAY 7
SUNDAY

What foods should I avoid forever?

The below foods have a deteriorating effect on a body and continued use may be the cause of future serious illness. Alcohol, cocoa, chocolate, commercial and oriental teas, all carbonated drinks, white flour products, cereals which have refined and bleached flour, commercial ice creams, all cakes and pies, roasted and salted nuts, white rice, black and white pepper, paprika, commercial candies, white sugar. Also stay away from any cheese that is pasteurized, aged less than six months or artificially colored.

Avoid fats and french fries and potato chips. Potatoes should be eaten very infrequently. Vary with sweet potatoes, which are more acceptable.

Avoid brown sugar, sugar syrups. Stay away from hollow foods such as commercial cookies, fast-food restaurant hamburgers or deep-fried fish.

BREAKFAST
1 fruit   1/2 grapefruit
1 toast   butter
Yogurt
Apple butter
2 Graham crackers
Herb tea or coffee

DINNER
Fresh vegetable salad
Corn muffins
Cup of vegetable broth
Unsalted crackers
Cottage cheese on slice of pineapple
Garden peas
2 slices vegetarian chicken
Sweet potatoes
Deborah's Delight *

SUPPER
Fresh green leafy salad
1 slice toast
Asparagus soup on fresh corn bread
Fresh fruit punch (6 ounces)
Fresh grapes
Herb tea

* See index for recipe.

> Soak granola overnight in skim milk in refrigerator for tomorrow's breakfast.

LOOKING AHEAD
Monday
Granola, corn bread, sauerkraut, vegetarian hot dogs, carrots, corn cake, orange juice, raisin pie, corn chips, green pea and celery soup.
Tuesday
Grapes, grits, eggs, vegetarian bacon, eggplant, potatoes, vegetarian chicken, peach Jello, Melba toast, vanilla pudding.

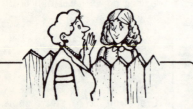

AUNT EFFIE...
How did Angus get rid of that scar?
One day Angus got into an argument. And a heated argument scorches both sides. As a young one, he had a chip on his shoulder. I told him a chip on the shoulder indicates that there is wood higher up. Well, he got hurt in the fight but I rubbed Vitamin E on the cut. No scar!

WEEK 3

Dr. Reams:
What are the symptoms of withdrawal when one is on a lemon water or water fast in a nutrition program? Does withdrawal involve having a temperature?

Some people will get a temperature. If you have a parasite in your system, you will have a temperature. Withdrawal is change of body chemistry from one pattern to another.

* * *

Dr. Reams:
Do vegetables have to be blanched, as we are told in cookbooks, before freezing?

No! Blanching ruins foods. Never blanch them. Cook them like you are going to serve them on the table and they retain their vitamins. But when you blanch them, they lose their vitamins. When you cook them, do not overcook them nor cook them with too much heat. Then you can freeze them and keep them for up to 2 years retaining most of their vitamin and mineral content.

* * *

Dr. Reams:
What about curry and nutmeg? Are they ok to use?

Some people can tolerate curry. To others it is like poison. Nutmeg is like the old fashioned black pepper. If you look at it under a microscope it looks like cut glass. You should not use nutmeg nor table pepper in your meal planning. Nutmeg and pepper only serve to aggravate a functioning body . . . like a thorn in the flesh. They can also cause bleeding of hemorrhoids.

> ... the pig, because it divides the hoof but does not chew the cud, it is unclean for you. You shall not eat of their flesh ... you may eat of all that are in the water, but anything that does not have fins and scales you shall not eat; it is unclean for you. *Deuteronomy 14:8-10*

WEEK 3   DAY 1

MONDAY

Why can't I eat pork products and shrimp, lobster, oysters and crab?

The Bible says these foods are unclean and you should not eat them. You may be living under grace but your bodies are the same that the Israelites had under law.

Pork, guinea pigs, rabbits, muskrat, snakes, catfish, tuna fish, lobsters, oysters, clams, shrimp, crabs, scallops and shellfish of any kind are unclean meats. (Yes, tuna fish is unclean. It is __not__ a scale fish)

These unclean meats release energy too quickly in your body. They digest so fast that you cannot use the proteins, which turn into urea and dump into the bloodstream so fast that the kidneys cannot eliminate them.

A urea build-up in the body ensues and excessive urea leads to many health problems.

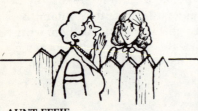

AUNT EFFIE ...
What can Sadie take for Psoriasis?

First thing ... stop worrying and start trusting God. Change her eating habits. Drink distilled water, 4 ounces every half hour. Unclog the colon. Take mineral supplements. Take two Lecithin capsules (1200 mg) daily. Apply liquid from another couple capsules right on the scaled areas.

BREAKFAST
1 fruit   banana
1 toast   butter
Granola
Tomato juice (4 ounces)
Herb tea or coffee

DINNER
Fresh vegetable salad
Corn bread
Sauerkraut and vegetarian hot dogs
Steamed carrot
Rebecca's Raisin pie *
Jerusalem Jumpers *
   (corn pancakes)
Orange juice (4 ounces)

SUPPER
Fresh green leafy salad
1 slice whole wheat toast
Green pea and celery soup
Corn chips
Yogurt
Carrot juice (6 ounces)

* See index for recipe.

   Soak grits tonight for tomorrow's breakfast.

LOOKING AHEAD
Tuesday
Grapes, grits, eggs, vegetarian bacon, eggplant, potatoes, vegetarian chicken, peach Jello, Melba toast, vanilla pudding.
Wednesday
Oranges, oatmeal, salad items, vegetable scallops, Hubbard or acorn squash, onion soup soufflé, apples, cranberry juice.

> A joyful heart is good medicine . . .
> Proverbs 17:22

WEEK 3 DAY 2
TUESDAY

What do you mean by "low stress" foods?

Low stress foods digest easily and quickly. They leave very little residue for the liver to detoxify. And, they do not cause toxic build-up in the colon or vascular system. Because low stress foods are more easily digested, they (a) offer their energy more readily to the body and (b) conserve energy that would otherwise be used in trying to digest high stress foods. Therefore, this energy can be used to increase energy reserves and increase endurance.

Low stress foods include: asparagus, beans, broccoli, Brussel sprouts, bell peppers, beets and beet tops, celery, cabbage, corn, cucumbers, cauliflower, endive, garlic, Jerusalem artichokes, kale, kohlrabi, mushrooms, onions, olives, okra, peas, pumpkin, romaine lettuce, radishes, rutabagas, sauerkraut, swiss chard, sweet peppers, squash, sweet potatoes, string beans, turnips and turnip tops.

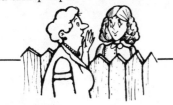

AUNT EFFIE . . .
Do you have a lotion for itches?
Yes. **Melt** together over hot water two tablespoons of lanolin plus one-half cup sesame seed or safflower oil. **Beat** in 3 ounces of witch hazel plus one tablespoon of liquid lecithin. **Take off heat** just as soon as mixture begins to thicken and turn bright yellow. Beat until well thickened. Apply daily.

BREAKFAST

1 fruit — grapes
1 toast — butter
Granny's Grits.
  Serve with raisins added as a cereal. See page 37 for recipe.
Scrambled eggs
Stripples (vegetarian bacon)
Herb tea or coffee

DINNER

Fresh vegetable salad
Corn bread
Esther's Eggplant casserole *
Baked potato (medium size)
2 slices of vegetarian chicken
Green drink *
Peach Jello
Hot or cold herb tea

SUPPER

Fresh green leafy salad
1 slice whole wheat toast
Vashti's vegetable soup *
Melba toast squares
Vanilla pudding
Grape juice (6 ounces)

* See index for recipe.

LOOKING AHEAD

Wednesday
Oranges, oatmeal, salad items, vegetable scallops, Hubbard or acorn squash, onion soup soufflé, apples, cranberry juice.

Thursday
Bananas, yogurt, tomato juice, corn muffins, corn crinkles, black-eyed peas, vegetarian turkey, corn on the cob, okra.

> ... do you not know that your body is a temple of the Holy Spirit who is in you, whom you have from God, and that you are not your own? For you have been bought with a price: therefore glorify God in your Body.
> *I Corinthians 6:19-20*

WEEK 3   DAY 3
WEDNESDAY

Should I steam my vegetables?

It is very beneficial to steam vegetables. Most Americans overcook vegetables and thus destroy the enzymes. Overcooking converts the starch to digestible carbohydrates and oxidizes the fat soluble vitamins minimizing their value. For vegetables to remain a low stress food they should be heated completely but remain crisp and chewy.

The crock pot or dutch oven are the easiest method of cooking. You will find that it is best to eat steamed vegetables at the evening meal. They are easier to digest. This also allows the stomach to empty before retiring.

The following vegetables are recommended for steaming: carrots, green beans, okra, parsnips, peas, pumpkin, red beets, rutabagas, squash, sweet potatoes and turnips.

Low stress dried fruits include: apricots, apples, currants, dates, figs, pears, prunes.

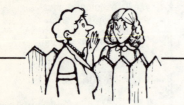

AUNT EFFIE...
Penelope has cold feet & leg cramps.

It's no wonder she don't cotton up to her husband! I take 400 units of Vitamin E, 600 mg. of Vitamin C, two Dolomite and four Calcium tablets daily. Gradually I worked up to 1000 units of Vitamin E daily. The diet did wonders for my legs. No more cold feet. No leg cramps at night.

BREAKFAST
1 fruit — orange
1 toast — butter
Oatmeal
  Sprinkle shredded coconut and raisins. Add a little vanilla flavoring.
Milk (6 ounces)
Herb tea or coffee

DINNER
Fresh vegetable salad
Corn bread
Hagar's Happening casserole *
Baked hubbard or acorn squash
Raisin molasses bars *
Hot or cold herb tea

SUPPER
Fresh green leafy salad
1 slice of whole wheat toast
Onion soup soufflé
Steamed carrot
Baked apple
Cranberry juice (6 ounces)

* See index for recipe.

LOOKING AHEAD

Thursday
Bananas, yogurt, tomato juice, corn muffins, corn crinkles, black eye peas, vegetarian turkey, corn on the cob, okra.

Friday
Oranges, oatmeal, salad items, chow mein, rice, cranberry juice, yogurt, bananas, meatless Irish stew and molasses cookies.

> ... if you will give earnest heed to the voice of the Lord your God, and do what is right in His sight, and give ear to His commandments ... I will put none of the diseases on you ... for I, the Lord, am your healer. *Exodus 15:26*

WEEK 3 DAY 4
THURSDAY

How can I determine what food combinations are best for me?

To some people, a low stress food may react as a high stress food. This may indicate an improperly functioning liver or an incorrect combining of foods.

Dr. Arthur F. Coca, M.D. writes extensively on how to check your body's adaptability to certain foods. His book, "The Pulse Test," suggests you take your pulse 30 minutes **before** eating. Then take your pulse again 30, 60 and 90 minutes **after** eating. If, after your meal, your pulse rate has not increased more than 10 beats per minute ... that food is considered low stress and non-toxic to you. If the pulse rate increases over 15 additional beats per minute, the food is high stress, it's poison to your system or you are allergic to it. It is best to plan your breakfast with vegetables and protein; your supper with vegetables and fruit. Vegetables act as a buffer.

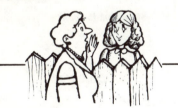

AUNT EFFIE ...
How's cousin Agatha's Asthma?

She tried all the drugs and had nothing to show but an empty bank account. Now she takes Vitamin A, Brewer's Yeast, B Multiples, 1500 units Vitamin C, 50 mg. Rutin, 400 units Vitamin D, 800 units Vitamin E, Lecithin, Sea Kelp plus 6 bone meal tablets, 3 garlic perles.

BREAKFAST
1 fruit — banana and orange
1 toast — butter
Baked apple — 1 yogurt
2 Graham crackers
Tomato juice (4 ounces)
Herb tea or coffee

DINNER
Fresh vegetable salad
Corn muffins — Corn chips
Cup of vegetable broth
Black-eyed peas on rice
Vegetarian turkey
Fresh corn on the cob
Steamed okra
Carrot juice (6 ounces)

SUPPER
1 slice whole wheat toast
Fresh green leafy salad
Solomon's celery soup *
Dried peach, apple Jello made in blender with skimmed milk and Knox gelatin
Grape juice (6 ounces)
Herb tea

* **See index for recipe.**
Prepare for Saturday's breakfast by soaking prunes (3 per person) for 48 hours in Lemon Water. Lemon Water is **one** part of fresh Lemon juice to **nine** parts of distilled water.

LOOKING AHEAD
Friday
Oranges, oatmeal, salad items, chow mein, rice, cranberry juice, yogurt, bananas, meatless Irish stew and molasses cookies.

Saturday
Rice, eggs, onions, vegetarian sausage, V-8 juice, prunes, yellow squash, sweet potatoes, vegetarian chicken, cauliflower.

> Beloved, I wish above all things that thou mayest prosper and be in health, even as thy soul prospereth. *3 John 2*

WEEK 3 DAY 5

FRIDAY

Doesn't the Bible say that no food is to be rejected if it is received with gratitude?

You are referring to 1 Timothy 1-5 which says that in the later times men will "...*advocate abstaining from foods*, ① *which God has created to be gratefully shared in by* ② *those who believe and know the truth*. For everything created by God is good, and nothing is to be rejected, if it is received with gratitude. For it is ③ *sanctified by means of the Word* of God and prayer."

① This phrase in the Greek reads, "...*which God has created for reception*." Not all meats were to be received during the Old Testament era. Leviticus 11 and Deuteronomy 14 spell this out very clearly.

② What was the truth that Paul was referring to? The "truth" was the true religion which encompasses that which is taught in both Old and New Testaments.

③ The Old Testament in Leviticus and Deuteronomy specifically indicate what foods were **not** sanctified by the Word of God during the Old Testament era.

God in Acts 10:9-17 and 15:20 revealed that with the death of Christ, the barrier between Jews and Gentiles was put aside and with it, the ceremonial food laws which went to support his barrier. The drinking of blood (and things strangled yet filled with blood) remained, however, barred.

Nevertheless, the dietary laws of Leviticus 11 and Deuteronomy 14, while not obligatory religiously to the Christian, contain wise advice for guiding a person's eating habits and choices of foods.

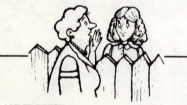

AUNT EFFIE...
What happened to Agatha's Arthritis?

She hung on to it as long as she could. Gave her something to talk about. Finally she accepted the fact that the pain wasn't worth the conversation. She cut her meat intake and increased her diet of raw foods. And she takes 12 Alfalfa tablets a day (4 at each meal). For her, it worked!

BREAKFAST

1 fruit	orange
1 toast	butter

Oatmeal with raisins
    Honey & allspice added to taste
Milk (6 ounces)
Herb tea or coffee

DINNER

Fresh vegetable salad
Corn muffin
Chicken Chow Mein on rice
Green beans
Boiled onion
1 yogurt
Cranberry juice (4 ounces)

SUPPER

Salad - leafy vegetable
1 banana
Eve's Meatless Stew *
Apple juice (6 ounces)
Corn chips
1 slice whole wheat toast
Herb tea

* See index for recipe.

LOOKING AHEAD

Saturday
Rice, eggs, onions, vegetarian sausage, V-8 juice, prunes, yellow squash, sweet potatoes, vegetarian chicken, cauliflower.

Sunday
Grapefruit, fruit salad, corn muffins, fish roe croquettes, turnip greens, zucchini squash, orange juice, tomatoes, mixed frozen vegetables.

> ... be sure not to eat the blood, for the blood is the life, and you shall not eat the life with the flesh. Abstain from blood and from things strangled ... Deuteronomy 12:23; Acts 15:29

WEEK 3 DAY 6
SATURDAY

Why can't I eat rare meat?

In several portions of the Bible we are told that the life of the flesh is in the blood and therefore we are not to eat the blood. Any disease an animal may have will defile the blood of that animal. The blood absorbs both the nutrients and the poison of the stomach and disseminates it. Most cattle today are killed by first stunning them with electricity or a blow to the head. After the heart stops, blood is drained out but most is still left in the animal. The meat weighs more because of this and you may believe it tastes better. But it can be harmful to your health!

Concerned Jewish people buy Kosher meats. Kosher meat is killed according to Scriptural principles and is more disease-free. Many related how after eating Kosher meat their stomach does not feel bloated or uncomfortably filled.

To drain the blood, soak meat in salty brine overnight in the refrigerator, then drain. Salty brine may be made by using 1/4 cup of plain salt to each quart of water. Soak in fresh water one day or more, changing the water frequently until all the blood is out. Drain and **cut off all fat.**

BREAKFAST

1 fruit	orange
1 toast	butter

Wilderness Wok *
Vegetarian sausage (2)
V-8 juice (4 ounces)
Phoebe's Prune Delight *
Herb tea or coffee

DINNER

Salem's Salad *
Corn bread
Fresh green beans
Yellow squash
Baked sweet potato
Vegetarian chicken (2 slices)
Egg Custard (served in cups)

SUPPER

1 slice whole wheat toast
Fresh green leafy salad
Cauliflower soufflé
Solomon's celery soup *
Yogurt
Apple juice (4 ounces)

* See index for recipe.

LOOKING AHEAD

Sunday
Grapefruit, fruit salad, corn muffins, fish roe, croquettes, turnip greens, zucchini squash, orange juice, tomatoes, mixed frozen vegetables.

Monday
Bananas, cracked wheat, chili, yellow squash, apple juice, dried peaches, prunes, apricots, Kirban cabbage soup, strawberry Jello, orange juice.

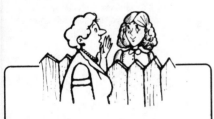

AUNT EFFIE ...
Did Angus get over Hemorrhoids?

Angus had quite a spell for a while. But they're done now. He took a combination of the following: Citrus Bioflavonoid Complex (100 mg.), Vitamin C Rose Hips (100 mg.), Hesperidin Complex (30 mg.) and Rutin (40 mg.). He took 12 a day and ate less meat.

> It is a perpetual statute throughout your generations in all your dwellings: you shall not eat any fat or any blood. *Leviticus 3:17*

WEEK 3 DAY 7
SUNDAY

Why can't I eat fat?

Over 1400 years ago, God gave the above dietary law to Moses. The advice is as good today as it was then.

All meats should be trimmed of fat. And meats should be broiled, baked, barbequed or stewed without fats or oils, **until well done**. When fats are heated by cooking, their composition is altered and the liver can not synthesize it. Therefore, the resulting cholesterol builds up in the arterial walls, breaks down and corrodes. Eventually that individual who is a consistent fat eater may develop arteriosclerosis (commonly called hardening of the arteries).

Fats didn't bother Eskimos because they ate raw seal and walrus blubber. But sophisticated man cooks his fat and this changes the health picture entirely!

Stay away from fried foods, french fries, doughnuts, pancakes, potato chips, popcorn and above all trim the fat from your meat!

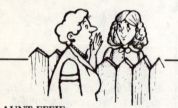

AUNT EFFIE...
Penelope's kidneys been acting up.

'Tain't no wonder, the way she eats. When Aunt Bertha got to jumping and hopping with shootin' pain, she took 300 mg. of magnesium oxide and 10 mg. of Vitamin B6 daily. She also got some kidney bean pod tea and drank 4 ounces every half hour. It didn't take long to put the fire out!

BREAKFAST
1 fruit — 1/2 grapefruit
1 toast — butter
Mixed fruit salad
Graham crackers (Two)
Herb tea or coffee

DINNER
Fresh vegetable salad
Corn muffins - add ginger
Fish roe croquette
Turnip greens
Zucchini squash halves
Sliced tomatoes
Sliced onions
Orange juice (6 ounces)

SUPPER
Fresh green leafy salad
1 slice whole wheat toast
Vegetarian vegetable soup
  Mixed frozen vegetables plus fresh celery and onions blended in blender - add a little potato buds
Yogurt
Cranberry juice (6 ounces)
Herb tea
Soak bulgur (cracked whole-grain wheat) overnight in distilled water for Monday's breakfast.

LOOKING AHEAD

Monday
Bananas, cracked wheat, chili, yellow squash, apple juice, dried peaches, prunes, apricots, Kirban cabbage soup, strawberry Jello, orange juice.

Tuesday
Cream of wheat, eggs, vegetarian bacon, yogurt, vegetarian meat balls and vegetarian spaghetti, Boston baked beans, onion mushroom soup, melon in season.

WEEK 4

Dr. Reams:
Which is better for constipation: flax meal or flax tea?

The meal is best because of its volume. Herb laxatives can be taken daily but you should try to correct your problem through eating properly. Gradually ease off dependence on herb laxative aids.

* * *

Dr. Reams:
What can be done for bad gas pains?

A colonic is the best thing I know. Also check your diet to see if you are eating nutritionally rich foods with sufficient roughage. If you are eating highly processed foods, cakes and pies and candy . . . then change your diet.

* * *

Dr. Reams:
Are vitamins an important part of your program?

What is a vitamin? Vitamins are enzymes. What is an enzyme? An enzyme is a product of a hormone. What is a hormone? A hormone is a living cell that is a product of an element or a mineral. Therefore, minerals are more important than vitamins! Without minerals we would not have any vitamins. Vitamins at their best are only a crutch. But when you need a crutch . . . you really need a crutch! And they are of great help to people regaining their health. But once you are healthy, you can dispense with them, if you can find them in your diet. If not, take supplements. But take minerals <u>with</u> meals. Take vitamins <u>between</u> meals.

> Rest in the Lord, and wait patiently for Him . . . those that wait upon the Lord, they shall inherit the earth. *Psalm 37:7, 9*

WEEK 4 DAY 1

MONDAY

What foods are "high stress" foods?

High stress foods include: all nuts (except almonds, boiled peanuts), alfalfa leaf, beef, black pepper, brewer's yeast, coffee, catsup, corn starch, crackers, cheese, chicken, eggs, fish, gravies, grapefruit, horse radish, honey in excess, sweetened fruits or juices, lamb, liver, limes, mustard, macaroni (except whole wheat), milk (Pasteurized), margarine, mayonnaise, organ meats, oriental teas, oranges, white potatoes, sugar syrups, soybean products, turkey, hardened shortenings and all white flour products.

High stress foods should **not** be a major part of your food intake. You will find that eating too many high stress foods robs your body of energy. The farther your body chemistry is from the perfect or normal Equation, the more energy will be lost. Plan your meals around **low stress** foods for better health.

BREAKFAST

1 fruit — banana or peach
1 toast — butter
Benjamin's Bulgur
  (Soak overnight, steam 1 hour. Season with vanilla or allspice.
Milk (6 ounces)
Coffee or herb tea

DINNER

Fresh vegetable salad
Corn bread
Chili man's chili
Corn chips
Yellow squash steamed whole
1 steamed carrot
Dried peach, dried prune and dried apricot soufflé
Apple juice (6 ounces)

SUPPER

1 slice whole wheat toast
Fresh leafy vegetable salad
Kirban's Cabbage Soup *
Corn chips
Strawberry Jello
Orange juice (6 ounces)

* See index for recipe

LOOKING AHEAD

Tuesday
Cream of wheat, eggs, vegetarian bacon, yogurt, vegetarian meat balls and vegetarian spaghetti, Boston baked beans, onion mushroom soup, melon in season.
Wednesday
Peaches, oatmeal, apple butter, corn muffins, vegetable scallops, lentil soup, molasses cookies, grape juice.

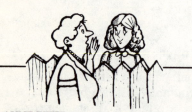

AUNT EFFIE . . .
Have you seen Bertha's Phlebitis?
A woman can be cured of almost any common illness by mentioning that the symptoms are signs of advancing age. Phlebitis, Aunt Bertha's inflammation of the veins, was quite troublesome. She changed her diet, took 600 units of Vitamin E daily along with 1000 units of Vitamin C. Now her legs are beauties!

> ...the Lord has anointed me to...bind up and heal the brokenhearted...to give a garland or diadem of beauty instead of ashes, the oil of joy instead of mourning, the mantle of praise instead of a spirit of fainting... *Isaiah 61:1, 3*

WEEK 4 DAY 2
TUESDAY

What beverages are acceptable?

First, the below beverages are **not** acceptable: cola drinks, coffee, commercial teas and juice "drinks."

Cola drinks of any kind are unacceptable because not only are they loaded with caffeine but a 6 ounce portion of a cola drink contains about 6 teaspoons of sugar. Sugar saps your energy!

Do not give up coffee or commercial teas overnight. Taper off slowly so your body can be accustomed to the change and the withdrawal will not be drastic.

Good coffee substitutes are: Pioneer, Kero, Postum. Good chocolate substitutes include: carob, cara-coa.

Acceptable teas include: mint teas, alfalfa tea, red or white clover tea, chamomile tea, chaparral tea, papaya and other herb teas. Other drinks are Loma Linda breakfast cup, blue violet.

Avoid fruit beverages that are labeled "drinks." These are mostly water, sugar and additives.

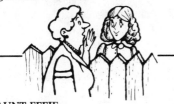

AUNT EFFIE...
Penelope's in Menopause!
Penelope has some diseases that haven't been invented yet! Doc Reams says "Menopause is a myth" and I believe him. Menopause is caused by a calcium deficiency. She needs a urine/saliva reading and calcium supplements. She should eat foods with high calcium content.

BREAKFAST
1 fruit   1/2 grapefruit
Pancakes   butter
Cream of wheat
Stripples (2) vegetarian bacon
Yogurt
Poached eggs (2)
Herb tea or coffee

DINNER
Fresh vegetable salad
Corn bread
Cup of vegetable broth
Vegetarian meatballs in vegetarian spaghetti
Boston baked beans
Carrot juice
Apricots (2) served on Graham crackers
Herb tea or coffee

SUPPER
1 slice whole wheat toast
Fresh leafy vegetable salad
Onion mushroom soup (Beat in one egg)
Honeydew melon (small slice)
Milk (6 ounces)

LOOKING AHEAD
Wednesday
Peaches, oatmeal, apple butter, corn muffins, vegetable scallops, lentil soup, molasses cookies, grape juice.
Thursday
Grapefruit, grits, eggs, V-8 juice, okra, carrots, orange juice, salad items, vegetarian Hungarian turkey soup, yogurt, apples.

> And on the seventh day God ended His work which He had made; and He rested on the seventh day. *Genesis 2:2*

WEEK 4 DAY 3
WEDNESDAY

Why am I a bundle of nerves?

Do you feel like a taut violin string in the morning . . . as though someone has plucked the string . . . and you vibrate all day on the edge of emotional exhaustion? You are not alone!

Could it be that you are violating one or more of God's laws? Most Americans do not know how to **relax**! (I mean really relax) To relax means to rest from worry and hard work.

Psalm 46:10 tells us to "Be still and know that I am God. . . ."

Many churches get their members so worked up in projects and committees that they neglect their family and their own well-being. They become nervous gnats flitting from one place to another trying to do God's work for Him.

Take a few minutes every day to do absolutely **NOTHING**. Rest on the seventh day. And let God take control. Believe me, He can handle it!

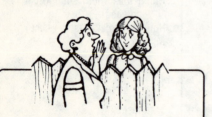

AUNT EFFIE . . .
Cora Mae's nails always split.

Not every woman in old slippers can manage to look like Cinderella. Cora Mae is more worried about her nails than her nutrition. Just chewing on sunflower seeds every day after lunch for a couple weeks ought to strengthen her nails as hard as anvils.

BREAKFAST
1 fruit   1/2 peach on Graham cracker
1 toast   butter
Oatmeal
  Add 1 egg for each 6 servings - raisins
Apple butter
Graham crackers (2)
Herb tea or coffee

DINNER
Fresh vegetable salad
Corn muffins - coconut added
Dorcas's Dream casserole *
Steamed carrot
Whole boiled onions
Grapefruit juice (6 ounces)
Banana strawberry Jello
  Made with strawberry jello and fresh bananas
Hot herb tea

SUPPER
1 slice whole wheat toast
Fresh vegetable salad
Jacob's Birthright Soup *
Corn chips
Grape juice (4 ounces)
Hot herb tea

* **See index for recipe.**
  Soak grits overnight tonight for tomorrow's breakfast.

LOOKING AHEAD

Thursday
Grapefruit, grits, eggs, V-8 juice, okra, carrots, orange juice, salad items, vegetarian Hungarian turkey soup, yogurt, apples.

Friday
Bananas, French toast, Maple syrup, Hush puppies, fish, sweet potatoes, Brussel sprouts, eggplant, fresh fruit cocktail.

> Better is a dish of vegetables where love is,
> Than a fattened ox and hatred with it.
> Proverbs 15:17

WEEK 4 DAY 4
THURSDAY

How should one eat?

Quietly, peacefully, without hustle or bustle! More dedicated Christians are sick because they break the cardinal rules of eating. They forget that they are feeding their body which is the Temple of the Holy Spirit. Here are some rules you should definitely follow:

1. **NEVER ARGUE AT THE DINNER TABLE**
   The dinner table is no time to discuss John's poor grades in Algebra or to complain to your wife that the meat is tough. **NEVER ARGUE!**
2. **TAKE THE PHONE OFF THE HOOK**
   <u>No</u> phone call is that urgent that it can't wait one-half hour ... not Helen's boyfriend nor your husband's boss ... <u>NOR</u> the President of the United States!

When you sit down to eat, plan to <u>RELAX</u>, get to know your family, enjoy wholesome food. And then, why not end the meal with family devotions!

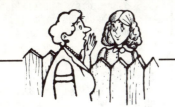

AUNT EFFIE ...
Fergus has a toe nail that's awful.
Old Fergus just don't mind me. Nail turned black with fungus problem. Then the nail thickened. What he should do is pierce Vitamin E capsules (400 I.U.) and apply it nightly on the toes for two weeks. He'll have the prettiest feet this side of Blue Ridge.

BREAKFAST

1 fruit — 1/2 grapefruit
1 toast — butter
Granny's Grits.
   Serve with raisins added as a cereal. See page 37 for recipe.
Egg omelette
Stripples (2) vegetarian bacon
V-8 juice (4 ounces)
Herb tea or coffee

DINNER

Fresh vegetable salad
Corn bread
Steamed okra
Steamed carrot
1 cup vegetable broth
Orange juice (4 ounces)
Hot tea

SUPPER

1 slice whole wheat toast
Fresh green leafy salad
Caleb's Carrot Soup *
Yogurt
Baked apple
Herb tea

* **See index for recipe.**

LOOKING AHEAD

Friday
Bananas, French toast, Maple syrup, Hush puppies, fish, sweet potatoes, Brussel sprouts, eggplant, fresh fruit cocktail.
Saturday
Pears, millet, Cream of Wheat, shredded wheat, graham crackers, green beans, turnip or mustard greens, carrots, Italian beans, apple juice.

> Is there no balm in Gilead; is there no physician there? why then is not the health of the daughter of my people recovered? *Jeremiah 8:22*

WEEK 4   DAY 5

FRIDAY

How can I find an inner peace?

In your purse or in your medicine cabinet you may have Valium or Librium or some other tranquilizer that gives you a false peace. It's a false peace for which you will pay a terrible price. Over 50 lines of side effects and warnings are listed in the pharmaceutical ads for these drugs! And these tranquilizers treat **no specific illness!**

Jeremiah witnessed Israel falling into sin. The scribes predicted all would be well (Jeremiah 8:8-12) but they lied. The harvest was ended and the Israelites had not prepared for the future. They had backslidden. There would be no balm ... no healing plant, no Great Physician as long as they disobeyed God. Jeremiah recognizes this fact. Read Jeremiah 9:1-7. Inner peace can only come through complete dependence on God. Beware of "scribes" who offer you peace in a pill!

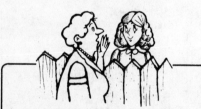

AUNT EFFIE ...
Did Angus have a Prostate problem?
You could always tell the time of night. Angus would get up 3 or 4 times a night. Finally, I put him wise. Take some zinc tablets and pumpkin seed oil every day, I told him. He finally minded me and now he can make it through the night. Changed his eating habits, too. Eats a fresh pear daily!

BREAKFAST
1 fruit   banana
1 toast   butter
French toast
Maple syrup
1 yogurt
Herb tea or coffee

DINNER
Fresh vegetable salad
Fish (any scaled fish)
Baked sweet potato
Brussels sprouts
Fresh fruit salad
Herb tea

SUPPER
1 slice whole wheat toast
Fresh green leafy salad
Elisheba's Eggplant Soup *
Corn chips
Fresh fruit cocktail
Milk (6 ounces)
Hot herb tea

* See index for recipe.

> See tomorrow's breakfast menu. Cereal Jubilee has to be soaked in skim milk in refrigerator.

LOOKING AHEAD
Saturday
Pears, millet, Cream of Wheat, shredded wheat, graham crackers, green beans, turnip or mustard greens, carrots, Italian beans, apple juice.
Sunday
Corn casserole, V-8 juice, corn bread, creamed corn, celery, onions, sweet potatoes, cranberry juice, vegetable noodle soup, corn crinkles.

Go up into Gilead and take balm ... in vain shalt thou use many medicines; for thou shalt not be cured. *Jeremiah 45:11*

WEEK 4 DAY 6
SATURDAY

What breakfast cereals are acceptable?

Commercial cereals loaded with sugar should be avoided. Learn to vary your breakfast meals. Do not eat the same thing each breakfast. Below are some cereals that are nutritious. But remember, dry cereals should be soaked in skim milk before you eat them. Otherwise, they will contribute to constipation.

Buckwheat, brown rice, cracked wheat, coarse ground grits, Farina, Loma Linda wheat germ, 3-minute Quaker Oats, Roman Meal, Kretschner wheat germ, Kelly's 14 Grain, millet and yellow cornmeal. Also Kellogg's or Nabisco 100% bran, shredded wheat or Cream of Wheat.

Bran is especially helpful for detoxifying and cleaning the colon. Most people start with 1 teaspoon of bran per meal each day and gradually are able to use 3 teaspoons per meal. Fresh fruits may be added to breakfast cereals. Dried fruits should be soaked overnight in distilled water before using.

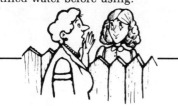

AUNT EFFIE ...
What is EDTA?

Hush, my child ... don't say that word around here. Stay away from EDTA. That's a food additive put in commercial salad dressings, sandwich spreads, soft drinks, beer and liquor. EDTA prevents the use by the body of much iron ... causes "hidden hunger."

BREAKFAST
1 fruit — pear or banana
1 toast — butter
Cereal Jubilee
  (Millet, shredded wheat, cream of wheat)
  First, cook millet. Add precooked cream of wheat. Add shredded wheat. Soak overnight in skim milk in refrigerator. Add honey and raisins.
Grape juice (4 ounces)
Peach (1/2) on Graham cracker
Herb tea or coffee

DINNER
Fresh vegetable salad
Corn bread — Green beans
Turnip or mustard greens
Steamed carrots — Onion soufflé
Orange juice (6 ounces)
Hot herb tea

SUPPER
1 slice whole wheat toast
Fresh green leafy salad
Solomon's celery soup *
Apple juice (4 ounces)
Peach (1/2) on Graham cracker
Hot herb tea
* See index for recipe.

LOOKING AHEAD
Sunday
Corn casserole, V-8 juice, corn bread, creamed corn, celery, onions, sweet potatoes, cranberry juice, vegetable noodle soup, corn crinkles.

Monday
Bananas, shredded wheat, cottage cheese, skim milk, corn muffins, corn on the cob, chicken a la king, pumpkin pie, Salem's Salad, yogurt shake.

> Cast thy burden upon the Lord, and He shall sustain thee: He shall never suffer the righteous to be shaken. *Psalm 55:22*

WEEK 4 DAY 7
SUNDAY

What fish and fowl can I eat?

Dr. Reams believes that acceptable meats of any kind should be eaten only 3 times a week. This would include fish and fowl in the 3-times quota (except if one is a heavy laborer).

Fish should not be cooked with fats or oils, but rather broiled, baked or boiled in stews. Acceptable fish include: anchovies, bass, bream, fresh water carp, cod, fish roe, flounder, haddock, mullet, perch, pike, red snapper, salmon, shad, sardines, trout etc.

Fish is the easiest meat to assimilate followed by chicken or turkey. It is better not to buy precut chickens, chicken parts. If you buy frozen turkeys, select a brand that is well-known and crossed state lines placing it under U.S. government inspection. Do not buy a chicken with the breast skin missing or with the breast skin loose.

It is best to skin your turkey or chicken before you cook it. Broil, bake or stew your chicken. Do not fry it. And do not eat the chicken or turkey skin. Be sure to drain the blood as per previously stated recommendations.

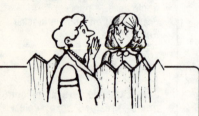

AUNT EFFIE . . .
Agatha's husband had a heart attack.
If I were Agatha, I would force feed her husband 800 I.U. of Vitamin E. He should take 400 I.U. before breakfast and another 400 I.U. between lunch and supper. I'd also make sure he drank 4 ounces of distilled water every one-half hour from 8 AM to 6 PM. He needs more salads, too.

BREAKFAST
1 fruit   1/2 grapefruit
1 toast   butter
Corn casserole with egg and onion
Pear (1/2) on Graham cracker
V-8 juice (4 ounces)
Herb tea or coffee

DINNER
Fresh vegetable salad
Corn bread
Green beans
Turnip greens
Yellow corn (creamed)
Celery - stuffed
Sliced onions and tomatoes
Sweet potato
Cup of vegetable broth
Cranberry juice (6 ounces)

SUPPER
1 slice of whole wheat toast
Fresh green leafy vegetable salad
Vashti's vegetable soup *
   Add vegetarian chicken squares
Raisin molasses bars *
Yogurt
Fresh fruit salad

* See index for recipe.

LOOKING AHEAD
Monday
Bananas, shredded wheat, cottage cheese, skim milk, corn muffins, corn on the cob, chicken a la king, pumpkin pie, Salem's Salad, yogurt shake.
Tuesday
Grapefruit, Cream of Wheat, eggs, salmon croquettes, spinach, whole pickled beets, Jello, oregano, corn crinkles, molasses cookies, yogurt.

WEEK 5

Dr. Reams:
What are the causes of overweight?

There are five causes of overweight.

1. An enlarged athlete's heart.
   You must keep your weight in proportion to the size of your heart.
2. A malfunctioning pancreas,
   in which it does not produce enough thyroxine for the thyroid gland to manufacture a substance to control the oils in your system.
3. Nervousness
   This can come from a lack of calcium in your diet or too much of the wrong kind of calciums. This causes nervousness and people become compulsive eaters.
4. Hereditary
   Check your ancestors. If they were large, stocky people, chances are you may follow their pattern.
5. Symptomatic obesity
   Less than 2% of people are overweight because of a basic genetic cause.

If when you are nervous and tense, instead of reaching for candy or strawberry shortcake or pie, try chewing on a stalk of celery or a carrot stick.

> ... put them all aside: anger, wrath, malice, slander, and abusive speech from your mouth.
> *Colossians 3:8*

WEEK 5 DAY 1
MONDAY

What about other meats?

Besides chicken, turkey and fish you have available veal, beef, lamb and organ meats. Beef and lamb are the most difficult for your body to assimilate.

Beef and lamb should be soaked in salt water overnight before cooking. Then drain and rinse making sure all blood has been drawn out. Cut off all fat. Beef and lamb should be cooked WELL. Do not eat rare meats. Make sure that the beef and lamb are well cooked to destroy any unwanted steroids and possible parasites.

If you eat organ meats, make sure they are fresh. Acceptable wild game are: Buffalo, Caribou, Deer, Goat, Moose, Pheasant, Quail and Squab. Squab should be soaked in salt water overnight and rinsed in morning.

Kosher meats, such as cold cuts, all-beef franks, lean corned beef are acceptable as are Shiloh, Worthington and similar brands.

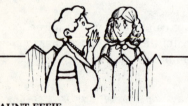

AUNT EFFIE...
Cora Mae's got the Flu again!
Cora Mae always has a virus and her kids always have runny noses. They should get off junk food, stop taking antibiotics every 5 minutes and start taking Vitamin C. Take 200 mg. every 2 hours for 8 hours. That's a lot better than taking 500 or 1000 mg. at one time.

BREAKFAST

Fruit — 1 banana
1 toast — butter
Shredded wheat
Cottage cheese served on 1/2 peach
Skim milk (6 ounces)
Herb tea or coffee

DINNER

Fresh vegetable salad
Corn muffins
Corn on the cob
Baked Beans
Chicken a la king on toast
Steamed onions
Pumpkin Pie
V-8 juice (6 ounces)
Herb tea

SUPPER

1 slice whole wheat toast
Salem's Salad *
Elisheba's Eggplant Soup *
Milk shake
Corn chips
Herb tea

* See index for recipe.

LOOKING AHEAD

Tuesday
Grapefruit, Cream of Wheat, eggs, salmon croquettes, spinach, whole pickled beets, Jello, oregano, corn crinkles, molases cookies, yogurt.

Wednesday
Pears, butter, oatmeal, crushed pineapple, vegetable scallops, parsnips, mushroom soup, salad items, corn crinkles, fruit cocktail.

> ... put on a heart of compassion, kindness, humility, gentleness and patience, bearing with one another, and forgiving each other ...
> Colossians 3:12, 13

WEEK 5   DAY 2
TUESDAY

What meat substitutes do you recommend?

First, don't let your tongue tell you what to do. More people die by wrong eating because they allow their tongue to dictate their eating habits. Learn to train your tongue to accept and like new wholesome foods.

The following meat substitues are both nutritious and easily digestible.

Loma Linda brand: Franks, Dinnercuts, Linketts, Nut Meats, Nuteena, Vegecuts.

Battle Creek brand: Nut Meats, Protose, Vegesteaks, Vegetable Scallops, Vegeburgers, Vegetarian Steak.

Worthington brand: Choplets, Franks, Linkettes, Sandwich Spread, Steakettes, Vegelinks.

Also recommended are Sunnydale Chicketts and Chili-Man's Friday Vegetarian Chili.

A suggestion: Be inventive. Try boiling Battle Creek Vegetable Scallops in Campbell's Mushroom soup. Other brands of meat substitutes found in health food stores may also prove acceptable to you.

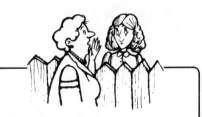

AUNT EFFIE ...
Agatha has a nervous stomach.

Agatha's stomach has been "fizzed" to death with all sorts of commercial concoctions. She takes every new thing she sees on TV. A cup of chamomile, catnip, comfrey or peppermint tea or some herb tea combination should make the churning waves a sea of calm.

BREAKFAST
Fruit   1/2 grapefruit
1 toast   butter
Cream of Wheat
    Add 1/4 can of cream style corn, plus 1 tablespoon Mazola oil
Scrambled eggs
Peach (1/2) on Graham cracker
Herb tea or coffee

DINNER
Fresh vegetable salad
Corn bread
Salmon Croquette
Spinach w/boiled egg
Sliced onion and tomatoes
Whole pickled beets
Jacob's Birthright Soup *
Corn chips
Jello
Herb tea

SUPPER
1 slice of whole wheat toast
Fresh green vegetable leafy salad
Tomato/onion soup
Dinah's Date Bars *
Yogurt
Homemade vanilla pudding
Fresh carrot juice (6 ounces)

* See index for recipe.

LOOKING AHEAD
Wednesday
Pears, butter, oatmeal, crushed pineapple, vegetable scallops, parsnips, mushroom soup, salad items, corn crinkles, fruit cocktail.

Thursday
Rice, eggs, onions, vegetarian bacon, apple butter, corn muffins, green beans, corn on the cob, okra, small potatoes, celery, eggplant, mushrooms, apple juice.

> And beyond all these things put on love, which is the perfect bond of unity. *Colossians 3:14*

WEEK 5 DAY 3
WEDNESDAY

What other foods are acceptable? The below food items are acceptable.

Breads
Bran muffins, rye crackers, rye bread, yellow cornmeal plus all other natural grain breads either leavened or unleavened.

Eggs
Two eggs twice a week (a total of 4 eggs) either boiled, poached or scrambled.

Fats
Olive oil or sesame oil, flax seed oil (cold pressed oils). Mazola or Fleischman's Oleo, 100% corn oil. Butter should be used sparingly and should not be subjected to high heats when cooking.

Milk
Skim milk and occasionally buttermilk, Yogurt, although a milk product is digested similar to meat and may be used 3-4 times a week.

Seasoning
Chives, pure cayenne pepper (red), cumin, garlic, herbs, kelp, laurel, marjoram, onion, oregano, parsley, sage, savory and thyme.

Sweets
Brown sorghum, carob, dextrose extract, unpasteurized dark honey, date sugar, maple sugar, black strap molasses, light or dark natural corn syrup.

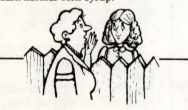

AUNT EFFIE...
Penelope has insomnia.

Penelope will never change her ways until the sun reverses its course and sets in the East. She stays up too late with her eyes glued to the "idiot lantern." She should take and run some lettuce through a juicer and drink the juice. She'll sleep like a baby.

BREAKFAST
1 fruit — pear
1 toast — butter
Oatmeal
  Add some honey, allspice, cinnamon.
  Add 1 teaspoon apple butter per serving
Crushed pineapple on 1 Graham cracker
Herb tea or coffee

DINNER
Fresh vegetable salad
Corn bread
Abishag's casserole *
1 sliced tomato, cucumber strips, ripe olives, sliced onions salad assortment
Herb tea

SUPPER
Salad
Caleb's Carrot Soup *
Corn chips
Fruit cocktail
Apple juice (4 ounces)

* See index for recipe.

LOOKING AHEAD
Thursday
Rice, eggs, onions, vegetarian bacon, apple butter, corn muffins, green beans, corn on the cob, okra, small potatoes, celery, eggplant, mushrooms, apple juice.

Friday
Bananas, vegetarian ham, vegetarian sausage, tomato juice, peppers, carrots, pickled beets, olives, green pea soup, carob chip cookies, yogurt, fresh grapes.

> The fear of the Lord is the beginning of knowledge: but fools despise wisdom and instruction. *Proverbs 1:7*

WEEK 5　DAY 4

THURSDAY

What may I expect if I fast?

Before you fast, you should check with your doctor. An important point to remember when you are fasting (or even on a light diet) is that you should rest. Complete rest is necessary if you expect your body to detoxify and to start to replenish its energy reserve.

Fasting is a flushing out process and as you flush out the toxins in your body you will experience withdrawal-type side effects. Some people go through a fast with flying colors, while others are miserable.

You may experience headaches. This is due to the ketone bodies and toxins building up in your system. With complete rest, these should flush out by drinking the proper liquids faithfully.

Some people experience a feeling of faintness for a brief period. Place a little honey on the tip of your tongue, keeping it in your mouth as long as possible and swallowing slowly. A little honey with your liquid intake is also helpful. Some notice numbness and tingling of their hands and feet. This is simply an indication that your sugar level is dropping. One should not get alarmed over this. Once the fast is completed, your taste buds will come alive. You will find it hard to realize that food could taste so good.

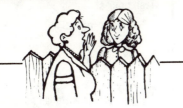

AUNT EFFIE...
What can I do for wrinkles?

The longest period in a woman's life is the 10 years between the time she is 39 and 40. Wrinkles are **not** a **normal** sign of old age. They are a sign you are encouraging illness through unbalanced body chemistry. Start drinking distilled water properly and 8 ounces of live vegetable juices daily.

BREAKFAST

1 fruit　　　　　1/2 grapefruit
Wilderness Wok *
Stripples (2) (vegetarian bacon)
Apple butter
Herb tea or coffee

DINNER

Fresh vegetable salad
Corn muffins
Cup of vegetable broth
Steamed green pole beans
Steamed corn on the cob
Steamed whole okra
2 small steamed potato with skins
Stuffed celery sticks
Herb tea

SUPPER

1 slice whole wheat toast
Fresh green leafy salad
Elisheba's Eggplant Soup *
Deborah's Delight *
Banana (1/2)
Pear (1/2)
Apple juice (4 ounces)

* See index for recipe.

LOOKING AHEAD

Friday
Bananas, vegetarian ham, vegetarian sausage, tomato juice, peppers, carrots, pickled beets, olives, green pea soup, carob chip cookies, yogurt, fresh grapes.
Saturday
Oranges, grits, vegetarian bacon, eggs, sliced pineapple, corn bread, Irish stew, apples, cranberry juice, orange juice.

> Trust in the Lord with all thine heart; and lean not unto thine own understanding. In all thy ways acknowledge Him, and He shall direct thy paths. *Proverbs 3:5-6*

WEEK 5 DAY 5
FRIDAY

What about frozen vegetable meats?

There are many acceptable brands of frozen vegetable meats in your health food store (and in some nutrition-wise supermarkets). Worthington, Loma Linda and Lange are all good brand names in this field.

Below is a list of Worthington Foods as a guideline:

Beef style (sliced), Chicken Style (Roll, Sliced or Diced), Corned Beef Style (Loaf or Sliced), Ham Style (Loaf or Sliced), Prosage (Pork Sausage flavor), Smoked Beef Style (Loaf or Sliced), Smoked Turkey Style (Sliced), Salisbury Steak Style and Stripples.

Prosage and Stripples would be cooked just as you would cook sausage or bacon.

Beginning your new diet, eat small servings to allow your digestive system to accept these new foods. Try using them in sandwiches with onions, lettuce, tomatoes and mayonnaise.

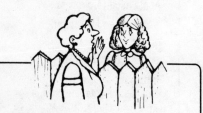

AUNT EFFIE . . .
Did you see Bertha's bloodshot eyes?
Look at your own eyes . . . closely. Do the whites of your eye resemble a Rand McNally road map? If so, you are sick! You are not drinking enough liquids. You are not eating the right foods nor getting the right rest. Your hospital is busy enough without your generating more business for them!

BREAKFAST
1 fruit — banana
2 toast — butter
Gideon's Gravy Gumbo *
Sausage (1) vegetarian
Tomato juice (4 ounces)
Herb tea or coffee

DINNER
Fresh vegetable salad
Corn bread
Stuffed peppers, baked
Steamed whole carrots
Whole small pickled beets
Ripe olives
Herb tea

SUPPER
1 slice whole wheat toast
Fresh green leafy salad
Green pea soup mixed with fresh celery blended and steamed for ½ hour
Carob chip cookies *
Yogurt
Fresh grapes

* See index for recipe.

Soak grits tonight for tomorrow's breakfast.

LOOKING AHEAD
Saturday
Oranges, grits, vegetarian bacon, eggs, sliced pineapple, corn bread, Irish stew, apples, cranberry juice, orange juice.
Sunday
Crushed pineapple Jello, Graham crackers, skim milk, vegetable salad, chicken a la king, onions, squash, spinach, coconut pineapple pudding, fruit salad, gingerbread cookies.

> Be not deceived; God is not mocked; for whatsoever a man soweth, that shall he also reap . . . he that soweth to his flesh shall of the flesh reap corruption. . .Galatians 6:7-8

WEEK 5 DAY 6
SATURDAY

What foods can I use in place of harsh, chemical laxatives?

America is the land of clogged colons. We are eating our way into the hospital. A majority of people include in their diet highly refined foods such as cakes, candies and pies . . . foods that provide no roughage for the colon and are nutrition-poor.

A teaspoon or two of bran on your cereal in the morning has proven beneficial. Gradually, work up to two or three teaspoons of bran at each meal.

Dr. Reams recommends a fresh pear in the morning, first thing upon rising. Or run the pear through your juicer and drink the juice.

Prune juice, upon arising, is also beneficial. Up to 180 pounds, drink 4 ounces every morning. If you are over 180 pounds, drink 6 ounces. If your sugar is high, you should drink the unsweetened prune juice.

Include in your diet sufficient raw vegetables and fruits to provide the natural roughage your system requires. Many nutritionists believe one or two movements a day is normal.

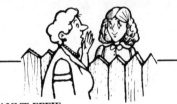

AUNT EFFIE . . .
Was Fergus ever impotent?

One time he was 'cause he junked up his system with hollow foods. I stuffed 1000 units of Vitamin E down his throat each morning with brewer's yeast and an 8 ounce carrot juice cocktail, combined with one pear. I made sure he only ate meat 3 times a week and drank distilled water every half hour. Things changed!

BREAKFAST
Fruit — 1 orange
1 toast — butter
Granny's Grits.
  Serve with raisins added as a cereal. See page 37 for recipe.
Stripples (2) — 1 boiled egg
1 pineapple slice on Graham cracker with 2 grapefruit sections
Herb tea or coffee

DINNER
Fresh vegetable salad
Corn bread
Eve's Meatless Stew *
  plus 1 beef cube per person
1 baked apple
Cranberry juice (6 ounces)
Sliced onions and beets

SUPPER
1 slice whole wheat toast
Fresh green leafy salad
Ream's Review Soup *
1 sliced pineapple on Graham cracker with cottage cheese
Orange juice (6 ounces)

* See index for recipe.

LOOKING AHEAD
Sunday
Crushed pineapple Jello, Graham crackers, skim milk, vegetable salad, chicken a la king, onions, squash, spinach, coconut pineapple pudding, fruit salad, gingerbread cookies.

Monday
Grapefruit, millet, yogurt, corn bread, whole grain corn, okra, black-eyed peas, rice, tomatoes, apples, tomato soup, corn crinkles, cottage cheese.

> The fruit of the Spirit is love, joy, peace, patience, kindness, goodness, faithfulness, gentleness, self-control ... *Galatians 5:22-23*

WEEK 5 DAY 7

SUNDAY

How do I make Green Drink?

Green Drink may be taken if your sugar reading is 5.50 or higher. It is best to drink at mid-morning.

Your Green Drink may be made from the following: Any edible green leaf, Beets, carrots, celery, endive, escarole, lettuce, mint, green beans, garden pea leaves, romaine, fresh green okra. The following may also be used but may cause some gas; Bell peppers, broccoli, cabbage, collards, cauliflower, cucumber, garlic, leeks, onions and onion tops and radishes.

For flavor, you may add the following: Apple juice, fresh apple (1 apple per quart), grape juice (unsweetened), tomato juice, yogurt, V-8 juice, lemon water, honey, pineapple juice or a fresh pear.

If 50-125 pounds .... drink 4 ounces
If 126-165 pounds .... drink 6 ounces
If 166 pounds or over   drink 8 ounces

It is important that Green Drink be consumed **immediately** after making to acquire full benefits from the nutrients.

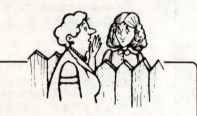

AUNT EFFIE...
What about frigidity?

Frigidity thrives in a tense or unhappy home life. It is triggered by our emotions. **First**, seek a deep, abiding faith in God. **Second**, learn to cast all your day to day burdens on Him. **Third**, approach life with a positive outlook. **Fourth** adapt good nutritional guidelines.

BREAKFAST

1 fruit   honeydew or orange
1 toast   butter
Crushed pineapple jello
Graham crackers (2)
Apple butter   Few grapes
Skim milk (6 ounces)
Herb tea or coffee

DINNER

Fresh vegetable salad
Corn muffins   Spanish rice
Chicken a la king
Steamed small onion soufflé
Steamed yellow squash
Spinach and boiled egg
Coconut pineapple pudding in serving cups
Fruit cocktail juice (4 ounces)
Hot herb tea

SUPPER

1 slice whole wheat toast
Fresh green leafy salad
Kirban's Cabbage Soup *
Fresh orange, grapefruit and crushed pineapple salad
Raisin Molasses Bars *
Hot herb tea

* See index for recipe.

LOOKING AHEAD

Monday
Grapefruit, millet, yogurt, corn bread, whole grain corn, okra, black-eyed peas, rice, tomatoes, apples, tomato soup, corn crinkles, cottage cheese.

Tuesday
Bananas, shredded wheat, skim milk, carrots, corn bread, peas, acorn squash, pickled beets, olives, date cookies, apricots, apples, yogurt.

WEEK 6

Dr. Reams:
Should one with low blood sugar fast?

If you have low blood sugar, you should not fast without supervision.

* * *

Dr. Reams:
Do you believe in acupuncture?

Acupuncture at its best only relieves pain. It does not remove the cause. It is important to use dietary methods to remove the underlying problem.

* * *

Dr. Reams:
Why do you recommend that raisins and many grains be soaked 48 hours before eating?

The soaking enables the grain or raisin to swell to its final size. In this way you eliminate gas and gas pains.

* * *

Dr. Reams:
What do you think of allspice?

I think it is fine to use allspice in your cooking. It is a beneficial spice.

> For who can eat and who can have enjoyment without God? For to a person who is good in His sight He has given wisdom and knowledge and joy ... *Ecclesiastes 2:25-26*

WEEK 6 DAY 1
MONDAY

Should I drink Carrot juice?

Carrot juice may be taken daily if your sugar reading is 5.49 or lower. In this 7 Week Diet Plan it is occasionally included. Some, where carrot juice is recommended daily, include in their carrot juice blend some spinach juice or celery juice. Others also put in a pear for the laxative benefits. The pear also acts as a natural sweetener.

If the carrot juice itself tastes bitter, then find a new source for carrots. Bitter tasting carrots are mineral-poor. Most health food stores carry carrots that are sweet and rich in nutrients.

Many believe that carrot juice is the most perfectly balanced vegetable juice available. It quickly releases its energy in your body. Its vitamin and mineral content helps the body to release energy from the stored fat.

Carrot juice should be consumed immediately after it is made. This assures you of the maximum in nutrients.

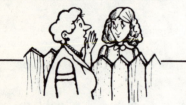

AUNT EFFIE ...
Poor Angus has such bad boils.
Angus don't pay no mind ... that's why. Like King Hezekiah, I made him mash a softened fig and tape it to the boil. Tonight I'm whipping up some red clover tea. He'll drink it twice a day. And I'll alternate with nettle tea the next day and sassafras tea the third day and repeat!

BREAKFAST
1 fruit   1/2 grapefruit
1 toast   butter
Ezekiel's Ecstasy *
Graham crackers (2)
1 yogurt
Herb tea or coffee

DINNER
Fresh vegetable salad
Corn bread
Corn (whole grain) - white and yellow
Okra soufflé
Black-eyed peas on rice
Sliced tomatoes
Stewed apples on Graham cracker
Hot herb tea

SUPPER
1 slice whole wheat toast
Fresh green leafy salad
Fresh tomato added to tomato soup half and half
Corn chips
Cottage cheese on pineapple slices
Herb tea
* See index for recipe.

LOOKING AHEAD
Tuesday
Bananas, shredded wheat, skim milk, carrots, corn bread, peas, acorn squash, pickled beets, olives, date cookies, apricots, apples, yogurt.
Wednesday
Cream of Wheat, vegetarian bacon, tomato juice, salad items, collard greens, fresh lima beans, vegetarian steak, yellow squash, Jello.

> Bless the Lord, O my soul, and forget not all his benefits . . . who satisfieth thy mouth with good things; so that thy youth is renewed like the eagle's. *Psalm 103:2, 5*

WEEK 6　DAY 2
TUESDAY

What other drinks does Dr. Carey Reams recommend?
Cranberry juice
Dr. Reams recommends cranberry juice for people whose body is not utilizing Vitamin C properly. If your sugar level is high (5.50 or above), drink it unsweetened. Best to drink cranberry juice in the early afternoon. The quantity you drink depends on your weight:

50 - 125 pounds	4 ounces
126 - 165 pounds	6 ounces
166 and up	8 ounces

Heinz Sweet Pickle Vinegar
Dr. Reams recommends Heinz Sweet Pickle Vinegar to help bring down high pH. Generally, one tablespoon three times a day. Why Heinz brand? Because this is the one brand Dr. Reams has tested that has been consistent in its quality and strength. You may also eat the pickles that come in the Heinz Sweet Pickle jar. Many find that the sweet pickle vinegar aids digestion and helps eliminate troublesome gas.

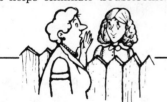

AUNT EFFIE . . .
Poor Penelope fears for diabetes!
Well, my granny used plain old blueberry leaves. A teaspoonful of dried cut blueberry leaves, steeped in a cup of hot water . . . drank it every 6 hours. She ate the berries too. Drank distilled water and took garlic perles. She placed more emphasis on raw foods. Kept the colon flowing!

BREAKFAST
1 fruit　　　　　　　　　　banana
1 toast　　　　　　　　　　butter
Hot shredded wheat with oatmeal and raisins
Skim milk (6 ounces)
Carrot juice (4 ounces)
Herb tea or coffee

DINNER
Fresh vegetable salad
Corn bread
Cup of vegetable broth
English peas
Baked acorn squash (1/2) filled with noodle soufflé
Steamed onions
Small pickled beets (3)
Whole ripe olives
Dinah's Date Bar *
　with 1/2 apricot
Herb tea

SUPPER
Salad, fresh vegetable
1 slice whole wheat toast
Vashti's Vegetable Soup *
Baked apple　　　　　　　Yogurt
Herb tea

* See index for recipe.

LOOKING AHEAD
Wednesday
Cream of Wheat, vegetarian bacon, tomato juice, salad items, collard greens, fresh lima beans, vegetarian steak, yellow squash, Jello.

Thursday
Apples, oatmeal, raisins, Graham crackers, vegetable scallops, eggs, corn, beets, onions, tomatoes, grapefruit juice, apple juice, fresh grapes.

> I am now eighty years old. Can I distinguish between good and bad? Or can your servant taste what I eat or what I drink? *2 Samuel 19:35*

WEEK 6 DAY 3
WEDNESDAY

What minerals does Dr. Reams recommend? Do elderly people benefit?

There are about 15 minerals in the Reams nutrition program. Of course, not all 15 are recommended to each individual. In the Scripture verse above, a wealthy Gileadite (near Jordan) whose name was Barzillai, brought provisions to David's army when David fled from Absalom. David invited Barzillai to come to live in the capital. Barzillai refused because of his age. He was old, perhaps showing the effects of hardening of the arteries and his taste buds could no longer distinguish flavors. Quite possibly his body chemistry was far from normal.

Thousands of elderly people, who have followed the Reams program of diet and mineral intake suddenly find they feel young again, their taste buds come alive.

It is true that any nutrition program which includes minerals and vitamins does cost money. To maintain health is costly . . . but to regain your health once you have lost it is far, far, far more costly! The choice is yours!

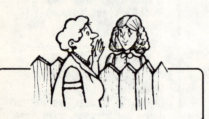

AUNT EFFIE . . .
Helen has morning sickness.

I never suffered from that. My mother, bless her heart, used to go out to the old peach tree, grab some leaves and brew up some delicious peach tea. It calmed my nerves, kept my colon unclogged and got rid of morning sickness. Of course, that's old fashioned.

BREAKFAST
Fruit 1 banana, peach or orange
1 toast   butter
Cream of wheat - served with
    boiled eggs
Stripples (2)
Tomato juice (4 ounces)
Graham crackers (2)
Apple butter
Herb tea or coffee

DINNER
Fresh vegetable salad
Corn muffins
Collard Greens
Fresh lima beans
Steaketts dipped in egg and onion
    batter (vegetarian steak)
Yellow squash (creamed)
Jello   boysenberry
Orange juice

SUPPER
Fresh green leafy salad
1 slice of whole wheat toast
Kirban's Cabbage Soup *
Yogurt   Corn chips
Jello   orange pineapple
Herb tea

* See index for recipe.

LOOKING AHEAD

Thursday
Apples, oatmeal, raisins, Graham crackers, vegetable scallops, eggs, corn, beets, onions, tomatoes, grapefruit juice, apple juice, fresh grapes.

Friday
Grapefruit, rice, onions, grape juice, carrots, corn meal, eggs, milk, fish, vegetarian sausage, baked beans, corn on the cob, apple Jello, celery, skim milk.

> Whenever you fast, do not put on a gloomy face as the hypocrites do . . . but you, when you fast, anoint your head, wash your face so that you may not be seen fasting by men, but by your Father who is in secret; and your Father who sees in secret will reward you openly.
> Matthew 6:16-18

WEEK 6 DAY 4
THURSDAY

How long should I take minerals?

Minerals and vitamins should **not** be taken during a fast or during an initial light diet program. Minerals and vitamin program should begin the day after the fast or end of your light diet period.

Initially, quite a few minerals and vitamins may be recommended by your Nutritionist. If you are faithful in taking these, within a month or two (because of noticeable improvement in your health), the quantity can be reduced greatly.

Algavim, a Reams' trade name mineral is generally recommended for use for an entire year . . . 2 capsules at each meal. The Reams' **Algavim** is a natural supplement of finely ground Norwegian kelp. It contains 60 minerals, Vitamins A through K, and amino acids.

Min-Col, a Reams' trade name mineral is recommended for the rest of your life. It is a natural, soft-rock mineral. It contains 66 elements in colloidal phosphate form.

These long term minerals not only help to restructure the body chemistry but they also maintain this normal balance and keep one's body from slipping back into its previous troublesome patterns.

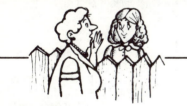

AUNT EFFIE . . .
I worry so every night.

Worry, honey, is like a rocking chair. You get plenty of exercise but it gets you nowhere. Lelord Kordel's granny used to say "The problems you face in the day ahead . . . will never be solved by worry in bed." Drink a lettuce juice cocktail and a gengsing capsule with a little honey and sleep well.

BREAKFAST
1 fruit — banana or peach
1 toast — butter
Oatmeal with cream style corn plus raisins, allspice, honey
Serve with skim milk
Tomato juice (4 ounces)
Graham crackers (2)
Herb tea or coffee

DINNER
Fresh vegetable salad
Corn bread
Hagar's Happening casserole *
Sliced beets
Sliced onions
   soak in ice water ½ hour before serving
Sliced ripe tomatoes
Yogurt
Grapefruit juice

SUPPER
Fresh green leafy salad
1 slice whole wheat toast
Soup of your choice
Fresh apple juice (4 ounces)
Fresh grapes
Herb tea

* See index for recipe.

LOOKING AHEAD
Friday
Grapefruit, rice, onions, grape juice, carrots, corn meal, eggs, milk, fish, vegetarian sausage, baked beans, corn on the cob, apple Jello, celery, skim milk.
Saturday
Pancake mix, pure maple syrup, grits, yogurt, creamed corn, tomatoes, cucumbers, Spanish rice, orange juice, corn crisps, grape juice, fresh fruit salad.

> If you forgive men for their transgressions, your heavenly Father will also forgive you. But if you do not forgive men, then your Father will not forgive your transgressions.
> Matthew 6:14-15

WEEK 6   DAY 5
FRIDAY

What about colonics and enemas?

Many years of poor nutrition often take their toll on the colon. Toxins build up, encrustations, impactions and other complications.

When the colon outflow is impaired, a flushing system plus good nutrition should prove beneficial.

A colonic must be administered by one who is licensed in this field. Your health food store can direct you to a trained colonic technician. The flushing procedure of a colonic does not overly distress the colon lining or the intestinal flora.

An enema, when recommended, can be done at home. Distilled water only should be used. You may wish to add the juice of one lemon. Do not use soap. The water bag should not be suspended more than 2 feet so that the water pressure is not too forceful. Introduce the water 3 times, trying to retain it 15 minutes each time, if possible. With the third evacuation, the water should be discharged fairly clear. Mineral supplements and yogurt help replenish the nutrients.

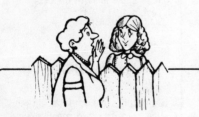

AUNT EFFIE ...
Penelope has high blood pressure.

She should relax. She has the most popular labor-saving device known today — a husband with money! I take two or three stalks of celery into a juicer with a couple carrots and a pear and drink it twice a day. And I take 3 garlic perles at every meal. Sometimes I drink cucumber juice, too.

BREAKFAST
1 fruit   1/2 grapefruit
1 toast   butter
Wilderness Wok *
Grape juice (6 ounces)
Carrot juice (4 ounces)
Herb tea or coffee

DINNER
Fresh vegetable salad
Hush puppies
Fish (any scaled fish)
Boston baked beans
   Fry vegetarian sausage until brown, then chop into small cubes and add to beans before baking
Corn on the cob
Raisin apple Jello
   made with Knox gelatin
Herb tea

SUPPER
Fresh leafy green salad
1 slice whole wheat toast
Solomon's Celery Soup *
Baked apple
Skim milk (6 ounces)
Herb tea

*** See index for recipe.**

LOOKING AHEAD
Saturday
Pancake mix, pure maple syrup, grits, yogurt, creamed corn, tomatoes, cucumbers, Spanish rice, orange juice, corn crisps, grape juice, fresh fruit salad.
Sunday
Pears, grapefruit, yogurt, corn bread, beans, yellow squash, vegetarian turkey, okra, potatoes, skim milk, carob chip cookies, vegetarian ham, celery, Jello.

> ... what does the Lord your God require from you, but to fear the Lord your God, to walk in all His ways and love Him, and to serve the Lord your God with all your heart and with all your soul. *Deuteronomy 10:12*

WEEK 6 DAY 6
SATURDAY

Can't I eat candies?

You should not eat commercial candies! Be inventive and bring your family together by making your own homemade candies. You can make delicious candies by grinding in a blender almost any dried fruits. Make a combination to suit your taste. Add a few ground nut meats, if you desire. Mold into balls. Roll in powdered milk or wheat germ. There's a wholesome nutritious snack.

If you like a chewy apricot candy . . . take 1/2 lb. dried apricots and soak them in water for 30 minutes. Then, to the apricots, **add** 1/2 lb. pitted dates, 1/4 cup honey and 1½ cups unsweetened coconut shreds. **Run** the dried fruits through a grinder. Gradually add the honey and the coconut shreds, mixing thoroughly. **Press** mixture into a 9-inch square pan, lightly oiled. **Remove** from refrigerator and cut into squares or bars. You will end up with 1¼ lbs. of delicious Apricot Chews!

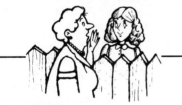

AUNT EFFIE . . .
I have such a sick headache.
Ben Franklin said, "Many dishes, many diseases, many medicines, few cures." Get that colon unclogged. I drink 4 ounces of distilled water every half hour from 8 AM to 6 PM plus juice cocktails and a little Thyme tea sometimes at night. I stay off cakes and candy.

BREAKFAST
1 fruit   apple
Jerusalem Jumpers *
Maple syrup
Egg omelette
Graham crackers (2)
Yogurt
Herb tea or coffee

DINNER
Fresh vegetable salad
Corn bread
Creamed corn (no meat) onion casserole
Sliced tomatoes and cucumber
Spinach and boiled egg
Spanish rice
Orange juice (6 ounces)

SUPPER
Fresh green leafy salad
1 slice whole wheat toast
Corn chips   Yogurt
Fresh onion soup
Grape juice (6 ounces)
Fresh fruit apple, pear, raisins and coconut salad
Graham crackers (2)

* See index for recipe.

LOOKING AHEAD
Sunday
Pears, grapefruit, yogurt, corn bread, beans, yellow squash, vegetarian turkey, okra, potatoes, skim milk, carob chip cookies, vegetarian ham, celery, Jello.
Monday
French toast, hominy, pineapple slices, corn muffins, peas, mushroom soup, hamburger, spinach, orange juice, salad items, yogurt, carrots.

> Search me, O God, and know my heart: try me, and know my thoughts: and see if there be any wicked way in me and lead me in the way everlasting. *Psalm 139:23-24*

WEEK 6　　DAY 7
SUNDAY

How much liquids should an individual take into his system every day?

Dr. Reams suggests:

1. Take your body weight.
2. Divide that body weight by two.

That is how much liquids, in ounces, you should drink daily. As an example, if you are 140 pounds. Divided by two is 70. You should be drinking 70 **ounces** of liquids daily.

Liquids should be taken **4 ounces** at a time; one-half hour apart. In other words, in a little over 8 hours . . . drinking 4 ounces every 1/2 hour, you will have taken your quota of liquids for the day.

Do not drink more than 4 ounces at each time. The body handles nicely the 4 ounce measurement. And by drinking distilled water (or other liquids) at 1/2 hour intervals you build a consistent body rhythm which should prove beneficial to one following a sound program of nutrition.

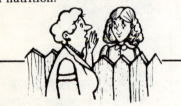

AUNT EFFIE . . .
Agatha has to get stronger glasses.

Ben Franklin said: "Keep your eyes wide open before marriage and half-shut afterwards." Agatha's nagging is her downfall. Glasses don't cure anything. They're a crutch. My dad used to grow Eyebright in his garden. We would drink it as tea. Health food stores carry it in capsule or pill form, too.

BREAKFAST
All fruit breakfast
1 pear, grapes and 1/2 grapefruit
1 or 2 cookies　　Yogurt
Hot herb tea

DINNER
Fresh vegetable salad
Corn bread
Cup of vegetable broth
Pole beans　　Yellow squash
2 slices vegetarian turkey
Steamed okra
Small boiled potato
Skim milk
　made into milk shake & chilled
Carob chip cookies *

SUPPER
Graham cracker
Corn chips
Fresh leafy green salad
Soup of your choice
　Add vegetarian ham or chicken, fresh celery. Cook celery well before adding to soup.
Carrot juice (4 ounces)
Fresh fruit jello

* See index for recipe.
LOOKING AHEAD
Monday
French toast, hominy, pineapple slices, corn muffins, peas, mushroom soup, hamburger, spinach, orange juice, salad items, yogurt, carrots.

Tuesday
Millet, eggs, vegetable salad items, asparagus, green beans, parsnips, onions, fresh fruit cup, pineapple juice, corn, apple dumplings, coconut.

WEEK 7

Some Food Guidelines:

1. Keep your meals simple. Do not have too great a variety of foods. There is a general tendency to overeat when you have too many choices.

2. Do not eat beans and potatoes together. Beans are heavy protein. Potatoes are heavy starch. Do not mix heavy proteins and heavy starches at the same meal. This results in fermentation and gas will drain you of energy.

3. Omit carbohydrates that are refined such as white flour products and refined sugar. Choose instead whole grain breads and natural sweet fruits (Try baking bread yourself. You will find it both relaxing and rewarding.)

4. Do not drink milk and eat meat at the same meal. In fact, it is best to eliminate milk from one's diet . . . other than skim milk.

5. Do not eat when you are emotionally upset or when you are overtired.

6. Try to eat more raw fruits and more raw fresh foods and less cooked foods. For a general guideline, at least 1/2 of the food you eat should be raw.

7. Most people tolerate fruit better if it is eaten by itself. As an example: if you are having a fruit platter, do not eat a hamburger with it. It is better, for one meal, simply to eat the fruit platter and not eat anything else at that meal. Watermelon and other melons are best eaten at least 2 hours after a meal and not with a meal. If your body chemistry is functioning properly a melon, in season, with breakfast is acceptable.

The above are general guidelines. Your body will let you know when you are eating the wrong kinds of foods or the wrong combinations.

> In the time of trouble He shall hide me in His pavilion; in the secret of His tabernacle shall He hide me; He shall set me up upon a rock.
> *Psalm 27:5*

WEEK 7 DAY 1
MONDAY

Should everyone drink Lemon Water? NO! Lemon juice is a high stress food. If the Sugar reading is 5.5 or above **or** if the sum total of Urea adds up to 26 or more . . . the lemon water combination should **not** be followed. (Lemon water is a combination of fresh lemon juice and distilled water) Taking lemon water with any of the above Equation factors would release too many toxins too fast in one's body. It could drive salts and urea into a danger zone. With such Equations distilled water only is recommended by Dr. Reams until the sugar or urea levels come down to more manageable levels.

Some people, upon drinking lemon water experience a burning sensation in their stomach. Such an experience generally indicates ulcers, Dr. Reams reports. He suggests, in place of lemon water in these circumstances, to substitute cabbage juice.

Juices should be prepared fresh and taken immediately after making.

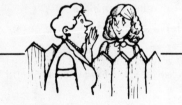

AUNT EFFIE . . .
Cora Mae's got this infection . . .
I don't know what's wrong with Cora Mae but maybe she hasn't discovered garlic. Garlic has a chemical called **allicin**. Its murder on unfriendly bacteria. It suffocates them. She should garlic up her salad, take garlic perles and don't kiss her husband.

BREAKFAST
1 pear or orange
French toast - maple syrup
Hominy with eggs and onions
Peach, pineapple, Graham cracker
Skim milk (6 ounces)
Hot herb tea

DINNER
Fresh vegetable salad
Corn muffins
English creole served on toast
  Hamburger, English peas, onions, mushroom soup, made into cream gravy. Brown hamburger in corn oil and add chopped onions just before hamburger browns. Then add English peas and mushroom.
Spinach and stuffed egg
Fresh orange juice (4 ounces)
Peach (1/2) on Graham cracker with cottage cheese

SUPPER
1 slice whole wheat toast
Fresh green leafy salad
Caleb's Carrot Soup *
Yogurt
Carrot juice (4 ounces)

* See index for recipe.

LOOKING AHEAD
Tuesday
Millet, eggs, vegetable salad items, asparagus, green beans, parsnips, onions, fresh fruit cup, pineapple juice, corn, apple dumplings, coconut.

Wednesday
Oranges, herb tea, apples, cauliflower, creamed corn, beets, vegetarian turkey, peach halves, cranberry juice, cabbage, corn crinkles, pineapple juice.

> I sought the Lord, and He answered me, And delivered me from all my fears. *Psalm 34:4*

WEEK 7 DAY 2
TUESDAY

What is the Lemon Water combination?

Lemon water is made with **fresh** (not reconstituted) lemons.

If under 120 pounds . . .
   3 ounces of fresh Lemon Juice is mixed with
  27 ounces of Distilled Water
    (Drink 3 ounces every hour)

If over 120 pounds . . .
   4 ounces of fresh Lemon juice is mixed with
  36 ounces of Distilled Water
    (Drink 4 ounces every hour)

The Lemon Water combination of 4 ounces is taken on the hour (8, 9, 10, 11, etc.). The 4 ounces of Distilled Water is taken on the half/hour (8:30, 9:30, 10:30, etc.).

Lemon water should **NOT** be taken without the advice of your doctor. Half your body weight (in ounces) is the amount of liquid one should take daily. A sweetener (honey, black strap molasses, etc.) should be put in the Lemon water combination. About 2 teaspoons per quart.

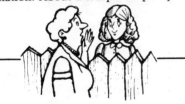

AUNT EFFIE . . .
Penelope has such a terrible cold.

Penelope spends more time on her face than she does what she puts into her body. Nature gives you the face you have at twenty. It is up to you to merit the face you have at 50. She should eat some raw onions at night . . . then slice some onions (or garlic) and put them in her socks when she goes to bed!

BREAKFAST

1 fruit   1/2 grapefruit
1 toast   butter
Ezekiel's Ecstasy *
  with 1 fried egg
Apple butter
Graham crackers (2)
Herb tea or coffee

DINNER

Fresh vegetable salad
Corn bread
Creamed asparagus on toast
Steamed carrots, green beans, parsnips, onions together in same container
Fresh fruit cup
Orange/pineapple juice (6 ounces)

SUPPER

Fresh green leafy salad
Corn casserole
Jacob's Birthright Soup *
Hard boiled egg
Apple dumpling with coconut
Carrot juice (4 ounces)

* See index for recipe.

LOOKING AHEAD

Wednesday
Oranges, herb tea, apples, cauliflower, creamed corn, beets, vegetarian turkey, peach halves, cranberry juice, cabbage, corn crinkles, pineapple juice.

Thursday
Bananas, vegetarian ham, celery, cucumbers, eggplant, green beans, strawberry Jello, orange juice, V-8 juice, salad items, molasses cookies, yogurt, apple juice.

> You will come to the grave in full vigor, like the stacking of grain in its season... Job lived 140 years... and Job died, an old man and full of days. *Job 5:26; 42:16-17*

WEEK 7　DAY 3

WEDNESDAY

How can I be free from nervous tension?

If you read the verse above very carefully, what the Bible is suggesting is that we should die **HEALTHY**! How many people do you know who have died sick?

The majority of illnesses that occur in our body occur because we have mistreated the Temple of the Holy Spirit. And as soon as illness occurs, we start pumping drugs into this Temple hoping to short circuit God's natural laws of healing.

Valium and other tranquilizers have become a way of life. They should not be! If you are nervous and tense because of day to day problems there are several things you can do. **First,** stop watching the 6 o'clock news on TV. It will only upset you. **Second,** RELAX. **Third,** examine very carefully your eating habits. Are you eating a lot of cakes, pies and pastry, fried foods and lobster, shrimp, pork, etc.? Then STOP EATING THEM and start eating wholesome, nourishing foods. **Fourth,** start drinking distilled water every half-hour from 8 AM to 6 PM daily. **Fifth,** chew on a stalk of celery every time you feel nervous. **Sixth,** drink carrot juice or green drink. **Seventh,** Seek God and exercise faith.

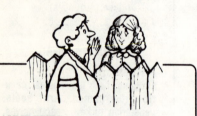

AUNT EFFIE...
Old Fergus's cholesterol's soaring!
Cholesterol charts aren't the whole story, Cora Mae. But I got a new diet for Fergus... an onion a day keeps the doctor away (and some of your best friends, too). Some strange things come out of an onion that seem to help folks with "old age" problems. Fergus and I just love onions!

BREAKFAST
1 fruit　　　　　　　　orange
1 toast　　　　　　　　butter
Baked apple
Graham crackers (2)
Yogurt
Skim milk (4 ounces)
Herb tea or coffee

DINNER
Fresh vegetable salad
Corn bread
Creamed cauliflower
Creamed onions, yellow corn
Red beets and sliced onions
2 slices vegetarian turkey entreé
Peach (1/2) on Graham cracker
　with cottage cheese
　　Shredded coconut on top
Cranberry juice (6 ounces)

SUPPER
Fresh leafy green salad
1 slice whole wheat toast
Kirban's Cabbage Soup *
1 fresh orange　　　Corn chips
Pineapple juice (6 ounces)

* See index for recipe.

LOOKING AHEAD

Thursday
Bananas, vegetarian ham, celery, cucumbers, eggplant, green beans, strawberry Jello, orange juice, V-8 juice, salad items, molasses cookies, yogurt, apple juice.

Friday
Skim milk, fresh fruit salad, mushrooms and mushroom soup, bell peppers, cream, sweet potato, onions, carrots, asparagus soup, salt-free corn chips, orange juice.

> Therefore shall a man leave his father and his mother, and shall cleave unto his wife: and they shall be one flesh ... Who can find a virtuous woman? For her price is far above rubies. *Genesis 2:24; Proverbs 31:10*

WEEK 7 DAY 4
THURSDAY

Will following a sound nutrition program bring joy back into my marriage?

There are many facets to a happy and successful marriage. They include: a mutual faith in God, a mutual respect for each other's desires, mutual goals and aspirations, a satisfying sexual fulfillment, a mutual understanding of each others problems.

Have you ever noticed on a rainy or cloudy day how people's dispositions change? They are generally gloomy, cranky and despondent. But when the sun shines, their whole attitude brightens.

Health has much the same effect. A person in poor health, or with a nutrition-poor body, is often hard to live with. The Bible says, in marriage, husband and wife become as one. But when a person is ill (and he may not realize he is ill), his interest or his ability sexually diminishes.

Many people on a junk food diet find themselves beset with such problems but don't recognize the fact that they are ill because of nutrition-poor eating habits. You may be pleasantly surprised at how your marriage suddenly comes alive when you start eating properly and drinking liquids faithfully!

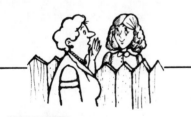

AUNT EFFIE ...
Are there blessings in a beehive?

Most certainly child. One of man's first supertonics was raw unstrained honey. Hay fever sufferers chew on honeycomb wax. Some tribes use honey royal jelly ointment to shrink hemorrhoids. Others claim it helps an enlarged prostate because it contains needed nutrients for this delicate area.

BREAKFAST
1 fruit — banana
1 toast — butter
Vegetarian ham omelette served on toast
Crushed pineapple on Graham cracker
Herb tea or coffee

DINNER
V-8 juice (6 ounces)
Fresh vegetable salad
Corn bread
Stuffed celery stick
Cucumber wedges
Sliced onions
Abishag's casserole *
Fresh green beans
Jello — strawberry
Orange juice (6 ounces)

SUPPER
Fresh leafy green salad
1 slice whole wheat toast
Creamed onion soup soufflé
  Add honey, blackstrap molasses, allspice
Corn chips — Yogurt
Apple juice (4 ounces)

* See index for recipe.

LOOKING AHEAD
Friday
Skim milk, fresh fruit salad, mushrooms and mushroom soup, bell peppers, cream, sweet potato, onions, carrots, asparagus soup, salt-free corn chips, orange juice.

Saturday
Pears, grape juice, melon, frozen peas, yellow squash, pickled beets, banana pudding, banana shake, skim milk.

> He that is slow to anger is better than the mighty; and he that ruleth his spirit than he that taketh a city. *Proverbs 16:32*

WEEK **7** DAY **5**

FRIDAY

How can you drink liquids every half-hour when you are travelling or working?

To maintain good health is sometimes a trifle inconvenient. But being ill or spending time in the hospital is a great deal more inconvenient!

Most people, when travelling on short one or two hour trips . . . fill several vitamin-type bottles with lemon water and distilled water. These bottles are generally 4 ounces. They carry a handy Memo Minder which sounds a bell at the half-hour interval . . . or they simply check the clock or listen to the radio for their time check.

If you are working, get into the habit of taking in a thermos of lemon water and distilled water and you will welcome the half hour "drink break." Others may think you a little queer but you will have the last laugh.

Drinking liquids every half hour will necessitate more trips to the bathroom . . . but that's better than a premature trip to the cemetery.

BREAKFAST
1 fruit   orange
1 toast   butter
V-8 juice (4 ounces)
Skim milk
Fresh fruit salad
Herb tea or cofffee

DINNER
Fresh vegetable salad
Corn muffins
Cup of vegetable broth
Dorcas's Dream casserole *
Baked sweet potato
Cold sliced beets and onions
Carrot juice (6 ounces)

SUPPER
Vegetable salad
Asparagus soup
Corn chips   Yogurt
1 slice whole wheat toast
Apricot pudding   Jello
Orange juice (4 ounces)

* **See index for recipe.**

> Prepare for Sunday's breakfast by soaking prunes (3 per person) for 48 hours in Lemon Water. Lemon Water is **one** part of fresh Lemon juice to **nine** parts of distilled water.

LOOKING AHEAD
Saturday
Pears, grape juice, melon, frozen peas, yellow squash, pickled beets, banana pudding, banana shake, skim milk.
Sunday
Oatmeal, fresh orange juice, corn bread, turnip greens, chicken a la king, yellow rice, sweet potatoes, Green drink, peach pie, avocado, carob chip cookies, carrots.

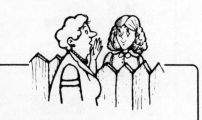

AUNT EFFIE . . .
What about royal jelly?

Royal jelly, Penelope, is the only food eaten by the queen bee. It is tremendously rich in pantothenic acid, biotin and nucleic acid. Fergus takes it for his gray hair and painful, burning feet. He says it helps his neuritis, too. It makes his bones stop aching.

> If any man among you seem to be religious, and bridleth not his tongue, but deceiveth his own heart, this man's religion is vain. *James 1:26*

WEEK 7 DAY 6
SATURDAY

How do you break a Fast?

You should not go back to regular eating habits the very first day after your fast. You should ease back slowly. If you fasted for one day, you should go on a light diet for the following day.

If you fast 3 days, you should take 3 additional days to ease back into routine. Below is a suggested diet after a 3 day fast.

First day
Eat an apple or a salad in the morning. Eat a salad and a piece of toast for dinner. Eat salad, soup and toast for supper.

Second day
Soak prunes, squeeze on some fresh lemon. And eat prunes along with soaking water for breakfast. Eat a salad, a vegetable soup and toast for dinner. Eat an apple at 2 PM. Eat a salad, a vegetable broth and a couple corn crinkles for supper.

Third day
Repeat the menu for the second day but add yogurt to breakfast. For dinner, include a boiled egg, a slice of whole-grain bread with butter. For supper, add a slice of cheese.

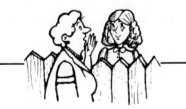

AUNT EFFIE . . .
Poor Bertha's arteries are clogged.

Most folk's got arteries that are lined with gunk. Fergus's dad used to put 2 teaspoons of honey, 1 tablespoon of lecithin granules and 2 teaspoons of safflower oil into a cup of fenugreek tea, stirring it well. He would drink 3 cups a day of this hot tea. All I know is he lived to a ripe old age.

BREAKFAST

1 fruit   pear
Muffin   butter
Fresh grape juice (4 ounces)
Honeydew melon or cantaloupe
Milk
Herb tea or coffee

DINNER

Fresh vegetable salad
Corn bread
Steamed carrots with frozen English peas
Creamed potatoes
Yellow squash
Cucumber wedges
Sliced onions
Whole pickled beets (2 or 3)
Rebecca's Raisin Pie *
Apple juice (6 ounces)

SUPPER

Fresh leafy green salad
1 slice whole wheat toast
1 small banana
1 fresh raw apple
Vegetable broth
Banana shake
    Concoct a milk shake with sliced bananas in blender

* See index for recipe.

LOOKING AHEAD

Sunday
Oatmeal, fresh orange juice, corn bread, turnip greens, chicken a la king, yellow rice, sweet potatoes, Green drink, peach pie, avocado, carob chip cookies, carrots.

> ... He which soweth sparingly shall reap also sparingly; and he which soweth bountifully shall reap also bountifully. 2 Corinthians 9:6

WEEK 7 DAY 7
SUNDAY

What is the key to good health?

The **first key** to good health is to become acquainted with your body. Find out why God put those parts there. Was the gall bladder installed so the surgeon would have a job? Does your body have a deficiency in Valium or Anacin or Sominex? Find out how your body is supposed to function. Most people know more about their car than they do of their own body (and they take far better care of their car!). Remember, you can trade in for a new car each year, but your body is the only one you are going to get. It can last 25 years, 35 years or 100 years depending on health maintenance.

The **second key** to good health is to provide your body with the fuel it needs to operate at maximum efficiency. Your body is the most complex system on earth! Yet, examine your eating habits. What are you throwing into this complex system? Fried foods, pork, cakes, pies, ice cream, pastry, white bread, alcohol, tobacco? The Bible says that **what you sow ... you will reap**. Start sowing wholesome foods into your body ... give your body the liquids that it requires to keep it flushing. If you sow bountifully ... you will reap bountifully in good health!

Following sound nutrition habits makes sense. But to many, adapting nutrition guidelines is just too simple. Most people look at those who speak out for sound nutrition as being unorthodox.

It is surprising at how many people, when they become ill, still will not radically change their diet. They would prefer to die **orthodox,** than to follow sound nutrition guidelines and live **unorthodox.**

BREAKFAST

Phoebe's Prune Delight *
1 fruit   pear
1 slice toast   butter
Oatmeal
   Add allspice or vanilla
Skim milk (6 ounces)
Herb tea or coffee

DINNER

Fresh vegetable salad
Corn bread
Turnip greens with egg
English peas - creamed
Chicken a la king on yellow rice
Baked sweet potato
Peach pie   **Green drink** *

SUPPER

Vegetable salad
1 slice whole wheat toast
Avocado (1/2)
Pinto bean and celery soup,
       mixed together
Carob chip cookies *
Yogurt
Carrot juice (6 ounces)

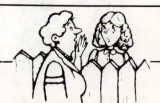

AUNT EFFIE ...
I'm going to miss you

Don't write my obituary yet. Death is nature's way of telling you to slow down. But I got lots more to tell you. Stay well. Remember, saying a prayer is not enough. You must live one, too. Start drinking distilled water and juice cocktails and let me know if you want Aunt Effie to keep writing.

INDEX

ABISHAG'S CASSEROLE, 26
Acne, 47
Acupuncture, 75
Additives, 42
Albumin, 40
Alcohol, 43, 50, 90
Algavim, 79
Allspice, 75
American Medical Association, 8
ANNA'S STEAMED DELIGHT, 30
Arteries, 89
Arthritis, 56
Asthma, 55

Beef, 68
Beef soup stock, 34
Beverages, 9, 35, 43, 50, 60, 61, 74, 76, 77, 82
Blanching, 51
Blood, 56
Boils, 76
Bonita, 43
Bowels, 12, 41, 47, 59, 73
Bran, 65
Breads, 70, 90
Brine, 57

CABBAGE SOUP, color insert
CALEB'S CARROT SOUP, 20
Cancer, 8
Candies, 59, 81, 90
Carbonated drinks, 50
CAROB CHIP COOKIES, 34
Carrots, 8, 10, 20, 73
Carrot juice, 76
Cause and effect, 45
Celery, 8, 10, 24
Cereals, 65
Cheese, 50, 60
Chicken, 66
Children, 43
Chocolate, 50
Coca, Dr. Arthur F., 55
Coffee, 9, 35, 60
Colon, 12, 41, 47, 65, 73, 78
Colonic, 59, 80
Comfrey, 37, 40
Constipation, 9, 59, 65, 73, 80
Cough, 37
Cranberry juice, 77
Curry, 51

DEBORAH'S DELIGHT COOKIES, 32

Diabetes, 77
Diarrhea, 9, 80
Digestion, 39
DINAH'S DATE BARS, 33
DORCAS'S DREAM CASSEROLE, 27

Eczema, 38
Eggs, 70
ELISHEBA'S EGGPLANT SOUP, 19
Enema, 80
ESTHER'S STUFFED EGGPLANT, color insert
EVE'S MEATLESS STEW, 28
EZEKIEL'S ECSTASY (Millet), 16

Fast, 43, 46, 51, 71, 89
Fat, 56, 57, 58, 66, 70
Fish, 9, 43, 52, 60
Flax, 59
Flu, 68, 85
Food combinations, 55, 83
Fowl, 66
Frigidity, 74
Fruit, 9, 73, 83, 89

Garlic, 84
Gas, 59
GIDEON'S GRAVY GUMBO, 29
Green Drink, 74

HAGAR'S HAPPENING CASSEROLE, 25
Hair, 88
Hands, dishpan, 45
Hay fever, 40, 87
Headaches, 81
Heart attack, 66
Hemorrhoids, 57, 87
High stress foods, 60
Honey, 60, 70, 71, 79, 85, 87

Ice cream, 50, 90
Illness, 44
Impotence, 73
Insomnia, 70, 79
Itching, 53

JACOB'S BIRTHRIGHT SOUP, 18
JERUSASLEM JUMPERS, 14
JUICE DELIGHT, 10
JUICE OF PEACE, 10

Kidneys, 58
KIRBAN'S CABBAGE SOUP, color insert

Kosher, 57, 68

Lamb, 68
Laxatives, 73
Lemons, 10, 42
Lemon water, 37, 41, 42, 47, 51, 84, **85**
Lettuce juice, 79
Liquids, 35, 50, 70, 74, 76, 77, 82, 88
Low stress foods, 53, 54

Meats, 43, 46, 56, 57, 68
Meat substitutes, 69, 72
Medicine, 12
Menopause, 61
Milk, 60, 70, 83
Min-Col, 79
Minerals, 12, 59, 78, 79
Morning sickness, 78

Nails, 62, 63
Nerves, 62
Neuritis, 88
Nutmeg, 51
Nuts, 50, 60

Onions, 85, 86
Overweight, 67

Pancakes, 14
Pears, 10, 73
Pepper, 50, 60, 70
Peppers, 46, 53
pH, 38
Phlebitis, 60
PHOEBE'S PRUNE DELIGHT, 17
Popcorn, 35
Pork, 52, 90
Potatoes, 43, 50, 83
Prostate, 64
Psoriasis, 52
Pulse test (Dr. Coca), 55

Raisins, 75
RAISIN MOLASSES BARS, 34
Raw foods, 47
Reams, Dr. Cary, 8, 34, 35, 37-41, 43-45, 51, 59, 67, 75, 77
REAMS' REVIEW SOUP, 34
REBEKAH'S RAISIN PIE, 31

SALEM'S SALAD, color insert
Salt, 39
Shellfish, 52
Shingles, 36
Sinus, 46
Sleep 70, 79
SOLOMON'S CELERY SOUP, 24
Steaming vegetables, 54
Stock, beef, 34
Sugar, 37, 50

Tea, 9, 35, 50, 60
Teas, herb, 61
Three-Day Diet, 9-12
Tuna, 43, 52

Ulcers, 44
Urea, 41
Urine/Saliva test, 8

VASHTI'S VEGETABLE SOUP, 21
Vinegar, 39, 77
Vitamin C, 38, 60, 68
Vitamin E, 36, 60, 63, 66, 73
Vitamins, 12, 59

Water, 10, 12, 35, 80, 81, 82, 88
WILDERNESS WOK, 15
Worms, 35
Wrinkles, 71

Yogurt, 80